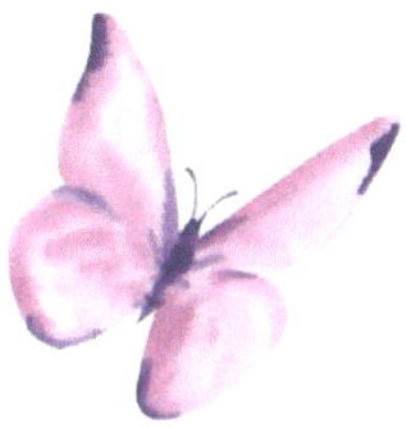

"You never know how strong you are, until being strong is your only choice."

- Bob Marley

NOURISHING TINY HUMANS: NEONATAL NUTRITION ESSENTIALS

STORM NUTRITION STUDY SUPPORT

ISBN # 979-8-9910953-0-3 *eBook/pdf;* ISBN# 979-8-9910953-1-0 *print*

Contents

NICU Levels

- All levels are capable of stabilization of ill or more preterm infants.

Level I:

Well Newborn Nursery

- Term or stable late-preterm infants
- (35-37 week GA)

Level II:

Special Care Nursery

- ≥32 weeks GA ≥1500g
- Moderately ill
- Some respiratory support

Level III:

NICU

- ≤32 weeks GA or ≤1500g birth weight
- Life-sustaining support
- Full respiratory support
- Advanced Imaging

Level IV:

Regional NICU

- Level III plus:
- Surgical Services
- Subspecialist
- Ped Anesthesiologists
- Transport
- Outreach education

Free Training Webinars and References

- ASPEN | Neonatal Care Resources (nutritioncare.org)
- https://pnce.org/ - start with overview of Koletzko guidelines
- Training Program in Neonatal Nutrition | ANHI
- Breastfeeding | ANHI
- NICU Nutrition 101 | 1 CPEU – Dietitians On Demand

Additional Recommended Resources

- Nutritional Care of Preterm Infants, 2nd Ed, 2021 (Koletzko)
- Pediatric Nutrition Reference Guide, Texas Children's Hospital
  - Pediatric Nutrition Reference Guide 13th Edition - Texas Children's Hospital (tchorderprocessing.com)
- Nutritional Strategies for the Very Low Birthweight Infant (Adamkin)
- Pocket Guide to Neonatal Nutrition (AND)
- Infant and Pediatric Feedings: Guidelines for Preparation of Human Milk and Formula in Health Care Facilities (AND)
- The ASPEN Pediatric Nutrition Support Handbook

Learning the Language

Preterm	Late Preterm	Term
< 37 weeks GA	34-37 weeks GA	38-40 weeks GA

Abbreviation	Definition
GA	Gestational Age – number of weeks post-conception
CGA	Corrected Gestational Age – age preterm infant would be if not born premature
Anthropometric Terms	
AGA	Appropriate for Gestation Age: 10th - 90th percentile at birth
LGA	Large for Gestation Age: > 90th percentile at birth
SGA	Small for Gestation Age: < 10th percentile at birth
LBW	Low Birth Weight: 1500 – 2000 grams at birth
VLBW	Very Low Birth Weight: 1000 – 1500 grams at birth
ELBW	Extremely Low Birth Weight: < 1000 grams at birth
FGR/IUGR	Fetal/Intrauterine Growth Restriction: fetal growth is less than expected in utero based on fetal monitoring/measurements; usually documented at birth
EUGR	Extrauterine Growth Restriction: traditionally defined as infant > 10th percentile at birth and < 10th percentile at discharge *(somewhat of a misnomer and term going out of practice)*
PNGF	Post-Natal Growth Failure – diagnosed when infant's weight is < 10th percentile at either discharge or 36-40 weeks CGA
HC	Head Circumference
Feeding Terms	
BF	Breastfeeding – infant is feed directly from maternal nipples
HM	Human Milk – any breast milk or fortifiers made exclusively from human milk, including maternal milk and donor milk products
MBM/MOM	Maternal Breast Milk/Mom's Own Milk – milk produced exclusively from infant's birth mother
EBM	Expressed Breast Milk – breast milk that is expressed via breast pump or hand pumping
EHMD	Exclusive Human Milk Diet – all milk and fortifiers are made from human milk; no bovine-based products provided
HMF	Human Milk Fortifier/Fortification – products used to provide supplemental kcal and protein to preterm infants; these may be from human milk or bovine-based (usually extensively hydrolyzed)
BBM/DBM	Banked Breast Milk/Donor Breast Milk – donor milk is collected and pooled to provide a homogenous human milk alternative when MOM is unavailable
HMBANA	Human Milk Banking Association of North America – accrediting organization for nonprofit human milk banks across US and Canada
HMOs	Human Milk Oligosaccarides – a group of complex prebiotic carbohydrates found naturally in maternal breast milk that are shown to support the infant microbiome and immune system
PTF	Preterm Formula – specially designed to meet increased energy and protein needs of preterm infant
Gavage	Orogastric feeding route

Baby-Friendly Hospital Initiative ©

To receive Baby-Friendly© designation, hospitals must follow The Ten Steps to Successful Breastfeeding and adhere to the International Code of Marketing of Breast-Milk Substitutes.
[Baby-Friendly USA ~ Upholding the Highest Standards of Infant Feeding Care (babyfriendlyusa.org)](babyfriendlyusa.org)

Summary of Principles:

- Encouragement of breastfeeding and rooming-in
- Avoid offering bottles and nipple feeding
- Marketing of formulas is prohibited, including offering of free samples
- Infant formula and feeding supplies required to be purchased at a fair market price

The Ten Steps to Successful Breastfeeding:

1. A) Comply fully with the International Code of Marketing of Breast milk Substitutes and relevant World Health Assembly resolutions.
1. B) Have a written infant feeding policy that is routinely communicated to staff and parents.
1. C) Establish ongoing monitoring and data-management systems.
2. Ensure that staff have sufficient knowledge, competence, and skills to support breastfeeding.
3. Discuss the importance and management of breastfeeding with pregnant women and their families.
4. Facilitate immediate and uninterrupted skin-to-skin contact and support mothers to initiate breastfeeding as soon as possible after birth.
5. Support mothers to initiate and maintain breastfeeding and manage common difficulties.
6. Do not provide breastfed newborns with any food or fluids other than breast milk, unless medically indicated.
7. Enable mothers and their infants to remain together and to practice rooming-in 24 hours a day.
8. Support mothers to recognize and respond to their infants' cues for feeding.
9. Counsel mothers on the use and risks of feeding bottles, artificial nipples (teats) and pacifiers.
10. Coordinate discharge so that parents and their infants have timely access to ongoing support and care.

The International Code of Marketing of Breast-Milk Substitutes

Provisions of the *International Code of Marketing of Breast-Milk Substitutes* require:

- No advertising of breast milk substitutes to families.
- No free samples or supplies in the health care system.
- No promotion of products through health care facilities, including no free or low-cost formula.
- No contact between marketing personnel and mothers.
- No gifts or personal samples to health workers.

- No words or pictures idealizing artificial feeding, including pictures of infants, on the labels or product.
- Information to health workers should be scientific and factual only.
- All information on artificial feeding, including labels, should explain the benefits of breastfeeding and the costs and hazards associated with artificial feeding.
- Unsuitable products should not be promoted for babies.
- All products should be of high quality and take account of the climate and storage conditions of the country where they are used.

Baby Friendly Application in NICU

- Encouragement of breast pumping with lactation support.
- Encouraged use of fortified human milk, including donor milk if appropriate.
- Promotion of skin-to-skin contact and family-centered care.
- Any breast milk substitutes, including special formulas, fortifiers, bottles, nipples, pacifiers and other infant feeding supplies, that are purchased by or for the NICU, are purchased at a fair market price.
- Does not restrict fortifier discharge programs for preterm infants.

Role of the NICU Dietitian

- Develop nutrition care plans based on assessment of intake, growth velocity and metabolic parameters.
- Provide diet education/recipe teaching for parents and caregivers.
- Collaborate on NICU formulary selection and feeding protocol based on emerging research and best practices.
- Collaborate on research and quality improvement projects.

Nutrition Screening for High-Risk Infants At Birth:

- Birth weight < 1500 grams
- Infants with IUGR or born SGA
- Alterations of GI tract or Signs of Feeding Intolerance

Estimated Screening for SGA in Mid- and Late-Preterm Infants

- Birth weight < 1500g @ 34 weeks GA
- Birth weight < 2000g @ 36 weeks GA
- Birth weight < 2500g @ 38 weeks GA
- Birth weight < 2800g @ 40 weeks GA/term

Infant Feeding Recommendations

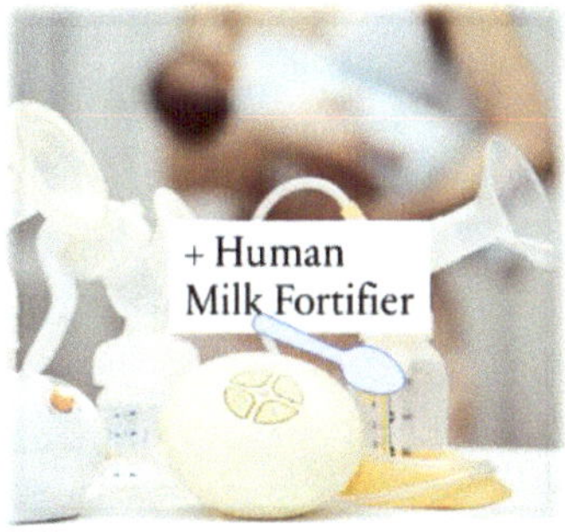

- Breast milk is gold standard – aka **"Liquid Gold".**
- Human milk fortifiers need to be added to breast milk in preterm infants.
- Preterm formulas contain less lactose, a combination of MCT/LCT, and higher protein than term formula (only LCT in term).
- Powdered infant formula should only be used when alternative sterile liquid products are not available.
  - Example: Elemental, semi-elemental, specialty formulas
- Upper limit osmolality to avoid tolerance issues is 460 mOsm/kg.

Importance of Human Breast Milk

- AAP recommends exclusive breastfeeding/use of expressed MBM (maternal breast milk) for the first 6 months, then in combination with age-appropriate foods until 12 months of age.
- Human milk provides beneficial enzymes, hormones, growth factors, antibodies, prebiotics, probiotics, and stem cells.

Benefits to Infant	Benefits to Mother
•Optimal, easily digested nutrition •Decreases risk for allergies and infections •Decreases risk of SIDS •Promotes healthy weight and decreases risk for chronic illness as adults •Increases cognitive development and early intelligence •Increases maternal-child bonding	•Burns 400 kcal/day and can aid in post-partum weight loss •Decreases risk of breast cancer •Decreases risk of obesity and chronic illnesses •Cost Effective •Increases maternal-child bonding

Strategies to Increase Use of Maternal Breast Milk

- Educate moms that breast milk is the optimal food for her baby and a therapy that only she can provide.
- Encourage moms to take infants to breast, hand-express, or pump within 1-2 (max 6) hours of delivery.
- Encourage mom to increase her fluid intake.
- Provide consistent messaging from all providers.
- Consult Lactation for maternal breastfeeding support.
- Consult Social Work to help moms acquire breast pumps and supplies if needed.

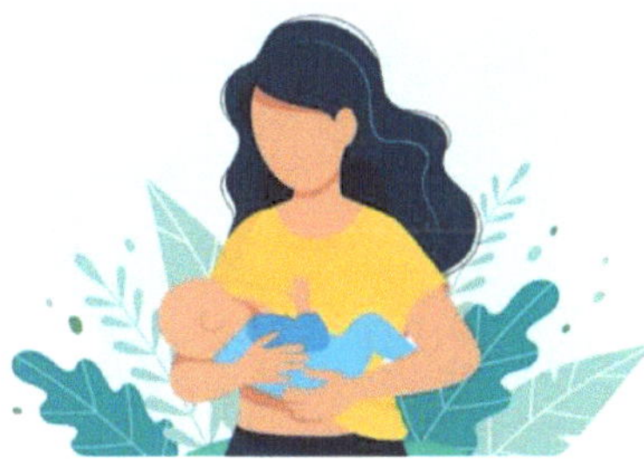

Feeding Recommendations by Maturity Level

Preterm	Fortified HM (10 ml HMF or Prolacta fortifiers) or Preterm formula (PE_{24} or SSC_{24}) PE = Premature Enfamil; SSC = Similac Special Care
Late Preterm	MBM with 5 ml HMF or Transitional formula (EnfaCare or Neosure)
Term	MBM or Term formula

Unique Needs of the Premature Infant

- Needs are increased nutrient to meet growth and development that would have been achieved in utero if delivered full term.
- Adequate growth is critical for optimal neurodevelopment, as the 3rd trimester is the most critical period for brain growth and development.
- Need to balance optimizing nutrition and neurodevelopment while minimizing long-term metabolic consequences associated with rapid catch-up growth.
- Appropriate protein and energy intake in the first 3 weeks of life is positively associated with optimal body composition in later life.
- Fortification of human milk is required to meet increased needs of prematurity.

Undernutrition

- Poor growth velocity and post-natal head growth are directly correlated with adverse neurodevelopmental outcomes.

Major contributing factor for development of BPD	Increased risk for retinopathy of prematurity (ROP)	Increased overall morbidity

Exclusive Human Milk Diet (EHMD)

- Definition: a diet composed of all human milk; with mom's own milk, donor milk, or both used the base feeding and fortified with human milk-based fortifiers.
- AAP recommends use of fortified human milk as standard of care in infants < 1500g.
    - HM fortification is essential for growth in preterm infants with high nutritional needs.
    - Infants receiving fortified HM have decreased morbidity and mortality, while maintaining desirable weight gain and providing cost-effective care.

Benefits of EHMD

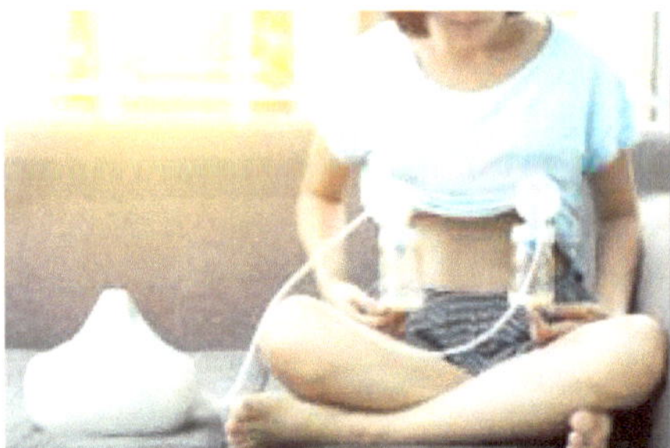

Optimal growth parameters and body composition	Improvement in feeding tolerance	Decreased risk of late onset sepsis, NEC, and BPD
Shorter hospital length of stay	Improved long-term developmental outcomes	Safe and cost-effective care

Composition of Human Breast Milk

- Breast milk composition is highly variable throughout the feeding, throughout the day, and throughout the stages of lactation from birth to weaning.
- Fat and lactose account for most of the energy in breast milk, which is on average 64 kcal per 100 ml or 19-20 kcal/oz.
- Feedings or expression starts high in carbohydrate and finishes high in fat to promote satiety for infant.
- Breast milk is highest in protein in the first 3 weeks of lactation and decreases significantly thereafter.
    - Early breast milk is estimated at 1.4 grams per 100 ml MBM.
    - After the first few weeks, protein content is widely variable, ranging anywhere from 0.6–1.1 grams per 100 ml MBM.

Use of Donor Breast Milk

- Donor breast milk donations often come from lactating mothers with a surplus of milk, so the milk donated can be diluted and lower in protein.
- Donor breast milk banks collect frozen milk donations, which are then screened for infectious disease and other factors, processed, pasteurized, and tested for presence of bacteria prior to distribution.
    - Milk from multiple donors is thawed in a refrigerator overnight, pooled, and mixed to ensure an even distribution of nutrients.
    - Following pasteurization, sample bottles are sent to an independent lab for testing.
- HMBANA is a non-profit organization and relies on volunteer donations, so donor milk is widely variable in nutrient composition.
- Prolacta and Ni-Q Human Donor Milk and fortification products are commercially processed with the ability to analyze products to provide consistent nutritional content.

Safety Considerations

- Fresh breast milk should be discarded or refrigerated within 4 hours of expression.
- Breast milk can be refrigerated for up to 24 hours or frozen for up to 12 months.
- Frozen breast milk can be thawed in a refrigerator or in a bowl of warm water.
- Thawed breast milk can be refrigerated for up to 24 hours but can only be at room temperature for 2 hours. It should never be refrozen.
- Breast milk should never be shared among mothers.

What is a Milk Lab or Formula Room?

It is a centralized feeding preparation area, staffed with technicians to prepare all human milk and formula products in a sterile environment for the NICU.

Photo credit: [Want to Build or Optimize Your Infant Feeding Prep Room? - Synova (synovaassociates.com)]

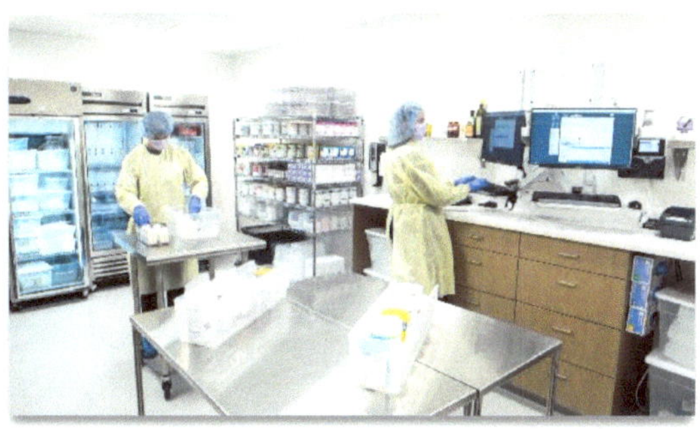

Initiation of Enteral Feeding

- Initiation of trophic EN (20 ml/kg/day) is recommended within 48 hours of life for infants who are not severely critically ill.
- Infants who are hemodynamically unstable on pressors or nitric oxide, have persistent bilious OG drainage, or abdominal distention should have feeding initiation deferred until stabilization is achieved.
- Early advancement to full enteral feeding volumes is recommended to promote optimal growth and body composition and does not increase risk of adverse outcomes.
- Starting EN day #4, feeding volume may be advanced by approximately 20-30 ml/kg/day if there are no signs of feeding intolerance and at the discretion of the Neonatologist.
- Infants < 750 grams may require slower initiation (15-25 ml/kg/day) and advancement of EN, as studies in extreme prematurity are limited.

Human Milk Fortification Options

Exclusive Human Milk Diet			
Prolacta +4	Prolacta +6	Prolacta +8	Prolacta Cream

↓

Bovine-Based Fortification	
Similac HMF • Hydrolyzed protein liquid concentrate • 1 packet per 25 ml HM	**Enfamil HMF** • Non-acidified hydrolyzed protein liquid concentrate • Available in standard protein and high protein • 5 ml HMF per 25 ml HM

Standard Fortification

- MBM or DBM is fortified with established amounts of HM-based fortifiers (Prolacta) or extensively hydrolyzed bovine-based fortifiers (Abbott or Mead Johnson) based on current weight.
- Fortification generally starts at 24-26 kcal/oz (+4 to +6 kcal/oz) and can be advanced as needed to meet target growth velocity up to +10 or 30 kcal/oz.
  - Use caution not to exceed 4.5 grams protein/kg.
  - Prolacta Cream is a fat modular product that can be utilized to add kcal without exceeding protein needs.
- In order to provide optimal nutrition for growth while the premature infant is advancing towards full feeding volume, it is recommended that fortification be initiated once the feeding volume is 60 ml/kg/day.

Sample of Standard Fortification Feeding Progression

Advancement of Enteral Nutrition & Fortification for Exclusive Human Milk Diet (EHMD):

Day of EN Feeding	Kcal/oz MBM or DHM	Feeding Volume (ml/kg/d)	Kcal/kg/d provided by EN	Protein g/kg/day provided by EN	PN Lipids (g/kg/d)
1	20	20	10-13	0.17-0.22	No change
2	20	20	10-13	0.17-0.22	No change
3	20	20	10-13	0.17-0.22	No change
4	20	40	27	0.44	No change
5	26 (PL+6)	60	55	1.5	Cut to 1/2 lipid[1]
6	28 (PL+6)	90	82	2.2	Off lipids [1]
7	28 (PL+6)	120[2]	108	2.9	0
8	28 (PL+6)	150[2]	137	3.7	0

[1]Both MBM & DBM contain 57.5% kcal from fat.

Up to 1/3 fat kcal can be lost to enteral tubing from mom's own milk, less with donor breast milk.

[2]If infant requires fluid restriction or if growth velocity does not meet goals, consult RD for consideration of PL+8.

Individualized/Targeted or Adjustable Fortification – Are They Practical Options?

- Both are shown to increase growth and promote lean body mass accretion with better feeding tolerance, improved metabolic profiles, and decreased morbidity.
- Both showed positive impact on body composition, linear growth, and head circumference.
- Very few NICUs (11.8% US survey respondents) are using human milk analysis and individualized fortification.
    - Barriers include cost, labor, and requirement for specially trained personnel.
- Adjustable fortification is recommended by the European Milk Bank Association as a more practical means to optimize nutrition.
    - This involves titrating modular protein supplementation on top of standard fortification based on BUN levels, which are monitored twice weekly.
        - If the level is <10 mg/dl, extra protein is added to the standard fortification.
        - If repeat level > 16 mg/dL, supplemental protein is decreased by 1 level of fortification.

Fortification method	Principle	Advantages disadvantages
1. Standard (STD) Fortification	Fortification method currently in use in most of the neonatal units. A fixed amount of fortifier is added to a fixed volume of HM according to the manufacturers' instructions.	Practical. But has not solved the problem of protein undernutrition for VLBW infants. Despite STD fortification many VLBW infants continue to have suboptimal growth.
2. Individualized HM Fortification Methods a. Adjustable (ADJ) Fortification	Protein adequacy is monitored by BUN twice weekly, cut-off levels of BUN are 10–16 mg/dl*. If the level is < 10 mg/dl extra protein is added to the STD fortification.	Practical, not labor intensive. Doesn't need expensive devices. Monitors protein intake of each infant. Safeguards also against excessive protein intake. Proven to be effective in optimizing growth and protein intake with a RCT. A real individualization method taking into consideration each infant's protein requirement.
b. Targeted Fortification	Macronutrient concentrations in HM are analyzed and based on the results milk is supplemented with extra protein and/or fat.	All macronutrients can be supplemented. Bedside HM analyzers are required. May be labor intensive. Supplementation is done according to the population recommendations, does not take into consideration that each individual infant's requirement may be different.

Arslanoglu et al 2019

*HM, human milk; VLBW, very low birth weight; BUN, blood urea nitrogen; RCT, randomized controlled trial. *BUN levels of 10–16 mg/dl correspond to blood urea concentrations of 21.40–34.24 mg/dl (3.57–5.71 mmol/l).*

Infant Formulas

**Note WIC requires minimum 20 kcal/oz*	**Caloric Density**	**Nutritional Differences**	**Examples**
Term Infant Formulas Designed to meet needs of term infant	19-20 kcal/oz*	Composition similar to breast milk Usually ~ 2 g protein/100 kcal	Similac Advance, Soy Isomil, Sensitive Enfamil, Gentlease, ProSobee (soy) Gerber Good Start, Gentle
Transitional Formulas Designed to meet needs of mid-late preterm infants or to transition from preterm to term formula	22 kcal/oz	Slightly increased in Calcium, Phos and Vit D. Higher protein, usually ~ 2.8 g protein/100 kcal	Neosure, Enfacare
Preterm Formulas Designed to meet high needs of preterm infants and match intrauterine nutrient accretion	20, 24, 30 kcal/oz (usually 24 kcal/oz)	Significantly increased in Calcium, Phos and Vit D High pro - ranges 3-3.3 g/100 kcal	Similac Special Care (SSC), Enfamil Premature (PE) (both also have high protein variations)
Hypoallergenic Or Amino Acid Based	20 kcal/oz	Often low in Vit D	Similac Alimentum, Nutramigen Elecare, PurAmino
Metabolic Formulas	Varies	Only available as powder; different formulas available for various inborn errors of metabolism	

Monitoring Feeding Tolerance

- Gastric Residual Monitoring:
    - A 2019 Cochrane review found no benefit to monitoring of gastric residuals to prevent NEC.
    - Gastric residuals are common in preterm infants due to shortened GI tract length, immature motility, and impaired digestion and absorption.
    - Infants on EN (10-20mL/kg/d) may have residuals of 50-100% due to normal gut secretion.
    - Residuals up to 2 mL for weight of 750g and 3 mL for weight of 750-1000g can be tolerated.
    - Routine monitoring of gastric residuals can increase interruptions in feeding that delay progression to full feeds, prolong exposure to parenteral nutrition and central venous access, and increase risk of extra-uterine growth restriction.
    - High residual is defined as residual > 25% or volume of 5mL/kg obtained in infants on larger feed volume (>75mL/kg/d).
- Abdominal girth increases of >2 cm from baseline over 12 hours could represent distention.
- The presence of bile in residual or emesis may indicate intolerance.
- If intolerance to MBM/fortifiers/standard formulas, try hypoallergenic formula before semi-elemental formula.

Assessing the Nutritional Needs of the Premature Infant

NUTRITION REQUIREMENTS					
	Kcal/kg	Protein g/kg	Calcium mg/kg/d	Phos mg/kg/d	Vit D IU/d
Preterm <1,000 grams	130-150	3.8-4.4	120-140	60-90	400-800
Preterm <34 weeks GA and > 1000 grams	115-130	3.5-4.0	120-140	60-90	400-800
Late Preterm 34-37 weeks GA	115-130	3.0-3.5	120-140	60-90	400-800
Term >38 weeks GA	100-120	2.0-2.5	200-1000 mg/d	100 mg/d	400-1000

Enteral Feeding Volume Goals

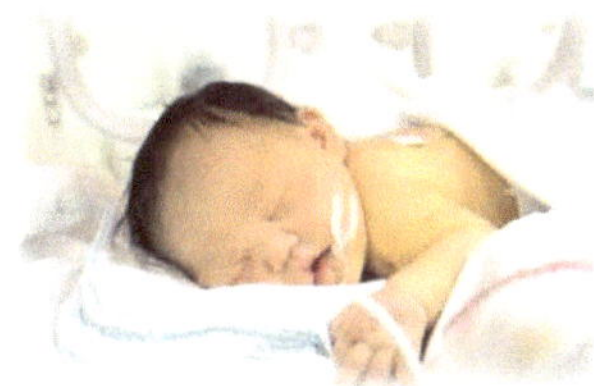

- <34 weeks CGA
    - 150 mL/kg/day preterm formula
    - 160 mL/kg/day fortified HM
    - 160-170 mL/kg/d transitional formula
- >34 weeks CGA: 160 mL/kg/d unfortified HM
- Restrict volume to 130 ml/kg/day for respiratory/cardiac issues.

Vitamin and Mineral Supplementation

Prolacta fortification does not include any vitamins in the product. In contrast, preterm formula and bovine HMF include vitamin supplements in the product. Babies on human milk and Prolacta need more vitamin and mineral supplements than those on formula or human milk with HMF.
Vitamins can be added once an infant reaches full feeding volumes.

- Poly-vi-Sol (PVS)
    - Contains Vitamins A, D, E and C, thiamin, riboflavin, niacin, vitamin B6, vitamin B12.
    - 1ml PVS contains 400 IU Vitamin D; does not contain Ca^{2+} or Phos.
    - Needed for all babies on unfortified HM, Prolacta-fortified HM, and transitional or term formula.
- Iron can be added separately or as PVS + iron once tolerating full feeds and PVS for 2 weeks.
- Vitamin D
    - Breastfed infants require a minimum 400 IU/day (1 ml) Vitamin D supplementation.
    - Babies with osteopenia or ALP > 800 will require an additional 400 IU (1 ml) of Vitamin D for total of 800 IU daily.
    - Vitamin D deficient Rickets – characterized by low or normal serum calcium, low or normal serum Phosphorous, high Alkaline Phosphorous, increased parathyroid hormone, and/or low 25 (OH) Vitamin D levels.
    - Calcium and Phosphorus
        - Unfortified human milk and term infant formulas are not adequate for preterm infants.
        - Steroids and diuretics interfere with Calcium and Vitamin D metabolism and can contribute to osteopenia.

Poly-vi-sol (PVS) & Vitamin D Supplementation Guidelines:

Feeding Regimen	Adjustment by Weight or Condition	Poly-vi-sol Supplementation	Vitamin D Supplementation
		Breast Milk	
BM w/ Prolacta	Wt < 2.5 kg	1 ml PVS	-
	Osteopenia or Alk Phos > 800	1 ml PVS	Add 1 ml (400 IU) Vitamin D *Increase to 1.5 ml (600 IU) if Vitamin D deficient*
BM w/ Bovine HMF	Wt < 2.5 kg	None	
	Osteopenia or Alk Phos > 800	-	Add 1 ml (400 IU) Vitamin D *Increase to 1.5 ml (600 IU) if Vitamin D deficient*
Unfortified BM	Wt <2.5 kg or SGA	1 ml PVS	-
	Wt > 2.5 kg	1 ml PVS w/ Fe	-
		Formula	
Preterm Formula	Wt < 2.5 kg	None	
	Osteopenia or Alk Phos > 800	-	Add 1 ml (400 IU) Vitamin D *Increase to 1.5 ml (600 IU) if Vitamin D deficient*
Transitional Formula	Wt < 5 kg	0.5 ml PVS w/ Fe	-
	Wt > 5 kg or Age > 6 months	None	
Term Formula	Wt < 3 kg	0.5 ml PVS w/ Fe	-

Reference: Pediatric Nutrition Reference Guide, 11th Edition, Texas Children's Hospital, 2016, page 67. Note: 1 ml PVS contains 400 IU Vitamin D

Additional Vitamin and Mineral Considerations in Prematurity

AquaADEKs	Vit A	NaCl	KCl
Fat-soluble vitamin given in PN-dependent babies	Used to help prevent/minimize BPD	Supplemented for preterm infants to support lean tissue growth	May be supplemented due to losses from steroids and diuretics

Sodium Supplementation

- Sodium content of fortified breast milk does not meet the increased needs for growth in preterm infants.
- Preterm infants are prone to increased Na losses due to immature kidney function and use of medications such as caffeine and diuretics.
- Sodium deficiency in premature infants is associated with increased morbidity, poor neurodevelopmental outcomes, and poor growth.
- Sodium supplementation may decrease the risk of late-onset sepsis and NEC.
- **Sodium Recommendations**
  - Sodium Requirements for preterm infants: 3 – 7 mEq/kg/day
  - ESPGHAN Recommendation: 3 – 5 mEq/kg/day
  - Maintain serum Na levels 136-140 mEq/L
  - Studies demonstrate improved weight gain by 20% in preterm infants given 3-5 mEq/kg/d Na supplements, started as early as DOL#4 for up to 5 weeks.

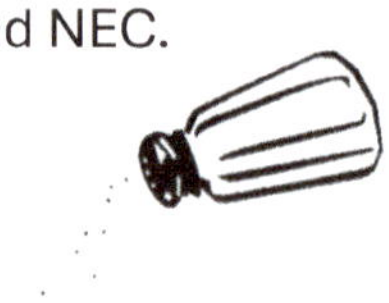

Zinc Supplementation

- Zinc is essential for cell proliferation, growth, and brain development.
- The greatest zinc accretion occurs in the 3rd trimester, so preterm infants often have negative zinc balance within the first 4-8 weeks of life.
- Preterm infants have a high demand for zinc due to rapid growth and increased losses due to immature kidneys and GI tract.
- Use of diuretics and steroids in CLD increase urinary zinc losses.
- Risk of deficiency is increased in SGA infants and intestinal failure.
- Signs of zinc deficiency include poor growth, diarrhea, rash, and immune dysfunction.
- Moderate zinc deficiency can increase the risk of NEC, CLD, and retinopathy.

Zinc supplementation has been shown to improve weight gain and linear growth velocity.

AAP recommended enteral zinc intake: 1.0-3.0 mg/kg/day.

Recommended parenteral zinc intake: 0.4 mg/kg/day.

Deficiency diagnosed as plasma zinc level ≤ 75 mcg/dL.

Feeding regimens for preterm infants (fortified MBM and preterm formulas) provide 1.2-2.0 mg/kg/day based on 120 kcal/kg/day caloric intake.

Supplemental zinc of 1 mg/kg/day elemental zinc (as liquid zinc acetate) for 2-4 weeks is indicated for zinc deficiency.

Supplemental zinc doses up to 4.5 mg/kg/day do not impact copper or Vitamin A absorption and retention.

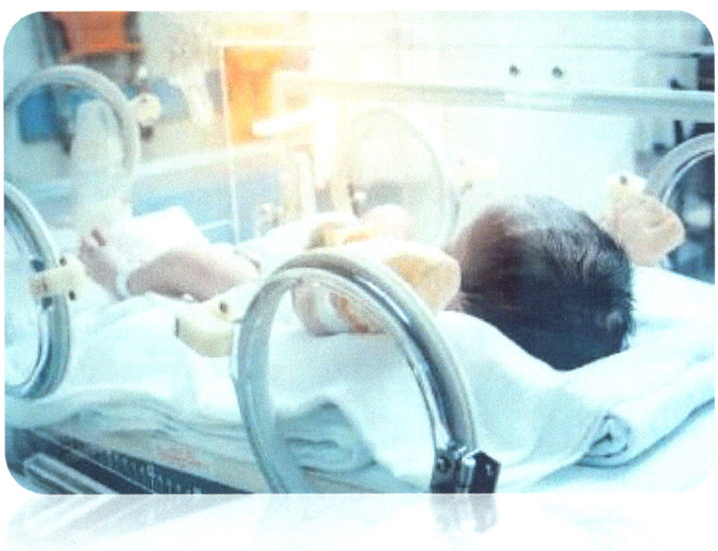

Laboratory Abnormalities

Consult NICU RD for recommendations if significant electrolyte abnormalities.

ALTERED LAB	POSSIBLE CAUSES	INTERVENTIONS
Hypoglycemia	• SGA or LGA • Syndrome of infant of diabetic mother • Hyperinsulinemia • Rapid discontinuation of IV dextrose	• Supplementation with IV dextrose • Continuous enteral feeds • Intermittent enteral feeds extended over 1-2 hours
High TGs (>300)	• Tolerance of lipid infusions is based on ability to hydrolyze IV fat • Infants < 33 weeks are slower to clear fat	• Decrease IL to 2g/kg/d initially; can decrease to 1 g/kg/d if persists • Not generally an issue or intervention with EN
High Phos	• Often transient as transitions off PN • >10 could indicate renal issues	• Does not require change in EN until > 10 • Use caution with low Phos feeds in preemies as cannot meet protein needs
High ALP	Osteopenia	If > 600 IU/L, add extra 1 ml Vitamin D (to reach 800 IU)
High Direct Bili	Cholestasis	Treatment of cause per Neonatology

Medications Impacting Nutritional Care

- Neoprofen, Indomethacin, and Tylenol are used to close PDA, and require infant to be NPO with TPN because these medications are known to decrease intestinal blood flow.
- Diuretics, specifically Lasix and Diuril, impair growth and cause K^+/Na losses.
- DART Therapy with Decadron is used to improve lung function in infants progressing to BPD/CLD and impairs growth.
    - Hydrocortisone is sometimes used for longer-term CLD steroids.
- Caffeine is used to aid in lung maturity/development.

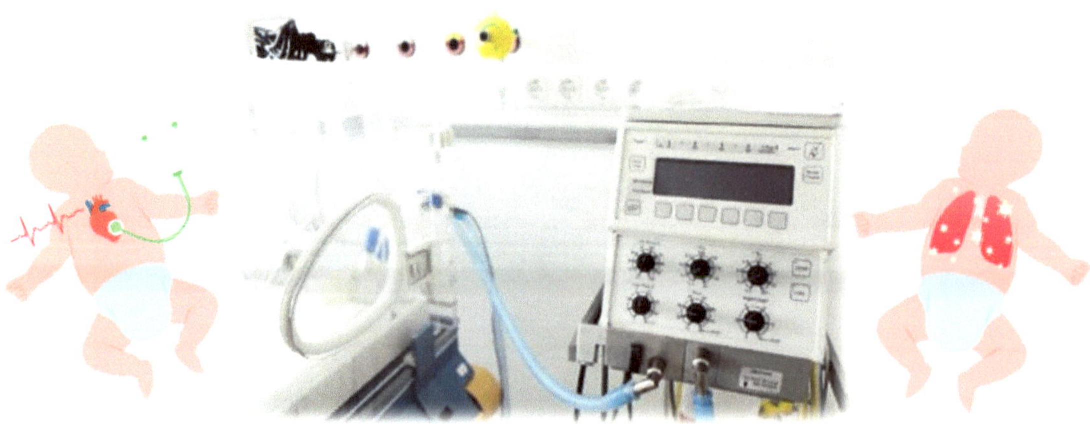

PN Support in Neonates

Indications for PN Support

- Parenteral nutrition is initiated as standard of care in premature infants when energy and nutrient needs cannot be safely provided immediately after birth and continues until needs can be met via enteral nutrition.
- "Starter" or "Stock" PN is immediately available at all hours and is generally used in the first 24 hours, but standardized PN is not recommended for routine care of preterm infants.

Severe Prematurity	Severe Critical Illness and/or ECMO therapy	Altered GI Structure or Function	Necrotizing Enterocolitis (NEC)	Late Onset Sepsis	Closure of Patent Ductus Arteriosis (PDA)

Timing for Initiation of Support

1st hours of life	**VLBW Neonates *(starter/stock PN)***
1-3 days	**Infants**
4-5 days	**Children and Adolescents**

Macronutrient Provision

- Neonates usually require 2-in-1 admixture with separate lipids over 12 hours.
- Consider SMOF lipids to limit inflammation associated with soy-based Intralipid.
- Minimum lipids to prevent EFAD, which can develop in as little as 2 days, is 0.5-1 g/kg/day.
- The maximum lipid infusion rate is 0.15 g/kg/hour.
- Maximum GIR (glucose infusion rate) for PN in infants is 14-18 mg/kg/minute.
- Neonatal PN contains increased taurine and tyrosine, which are essential amino acids in neonates due to enzyme immaturity.
- Cysteine is an essential AA in neonates, but it must be added to PN separately due to solubility concerns.

Needs Adjustment for Exclusive PN Support

Energy Needs	Initial PN: 50-60 kcal/kg/day
	Growth PN: 90-110 kcal/kg/day
Protein Needs	Initial PN: 2-3 g/kg/day
	Preterm Growth PN: 3.5-4.5 g/kg/day
	Term Growth PN: 2.5-3.0 g/kg/day
	Surgery: 2-3 g/kg/day

TPN CALCULATIONS *(sample calculation)*

Hyperalimentation:
Total Glucose Concentration (%) = 10
Total Protein (grams/kg/day) = 3.5
Total Fat (grams/kg/day) = 3

Glucose 10% @ 3.3 ml/hr
3.3 ml/hr x 24 hrs = 79.0 ml
79.2 ml x 10% (0.10) = 7.9 x 3.4 kcal/g = 26.86 kcal
26.86 kcal /wt (kg) 3.135 = 8.6 kcal/kg
Protein 3.5g/kg/d = 14 kcal/kg (4kcal/g)
Fat (IL) usually 3g/kg/d = 27 kcal/kg (9 kcal/g)

PN Electrolyte Dosing

Component	Preterm Neonates	Term Infants
Sodium	2-5 mEq/kg/day	
Potassium	2-4 mEq/kg/day	
Calcium	2-4 mEq/kg/day	0.5-4 mEq/kg/day
Phosphorus	Kg/day1-2 mmol/	0.5-2 mmol/kg/day
Magnesium	0.3-0.5 mEq/kg/day	

Potassium is left out of TPN on DOL#1 because kidneys are underdeveloped and do not filter it well.
It should not be added until kidney function is established.

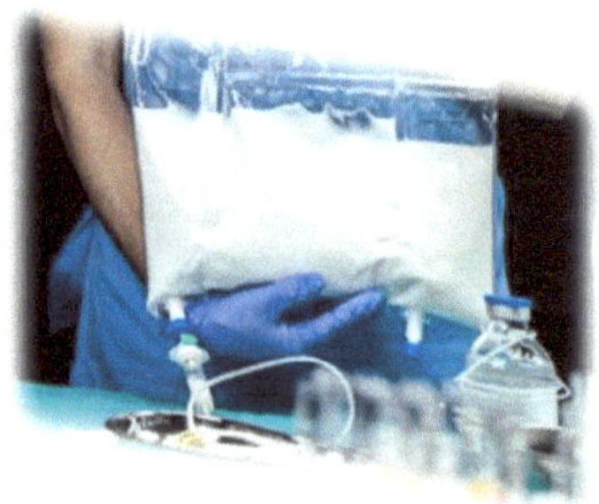

PN Vitamin Dosage

- <2.5 kg → give 2 ml/day
- >2.5 kg → give 5 ml/day

PN Trace Element Dosage

TE	***Preterm Neonates** (<3 kg)*	***Term Infants** (3-10 kg)*
Zinc	400 mcg/kg/day	50-250 mcg/kg/day
Copper	20 mcg/kg/day	
*Manganese**	1 mcg/kg/day	
*Chromium**	0.0006 mcg/kg/day	0.0006-0.012 mcg/kg/day
Selenium	1.5-2 mcg/kg/day	2 mcg/kg/day

**Recent recommendations indicate removal from neonatal PN.*

- Carnitine deficiency in infants or children on PN can cause brain abnormalities or neurological symptoms.
    - Dose of 20 mg/kg/day is recommended in long term PN.

Transition from PN to EN Support

- An average length of weaning from PN to full EN of 7 days is supported by current literature.
- EN should transition to the predominant feeding modality with decreasing PN as enteral volume reaches 80 ml/kg/day.
- Recommendation for target protein provision during the transitional period is 3.5 g/kg/day from combined feedings, with 1-2 g/kg/day provided as parenteral amino acids.

ASPEN Guidelines for Parenteral Nutrition in Preterm Infants

Initiate prompt initiation of PN after birth as soon as appropriate vascular access is obtained.

Protein recommendation: initial dose at minimum of 3.0 g/kg, with daily dose not to exceed 3.5 g/kg/day.

Higher protein doses may cause harm and evidence to support improved growth or neurodevelopmental outcomes is limited.

Daily advancement of lipids to target 3.0 g/kg/day to improve growth and decrease risk of EFAD or adverse outcome.

Either soy-based or multicomponent ILE can be used with careful attention to ensuring sufficient provision to prevent EFAD. No evidence that specific ILE composition enhances growth.

Avoid reducing dose of macronutrients for the purposes of preventing PNALD.

No evidence that specific ILE composition reduces PNALD risk or levels of unbound bilirubin.

Recommend against ILE dose reduction to prevent sepsis.

Micronutrient provision, including calcium and phosphorus, should be prescribed according to ASPEN/ESPGHAN consensus recommedations.

Premade PN "starter" or "stock" solutions should be provided for the first 24 hours after birth, but should not be used for routine care in preterm infants.

Routine insulin should not be used to for the purposes of improving growth outcomes in hospitalized preterm infants.

Neonatal Growth

Weight Change:

Infants normally lose 8-15% of birth weight in the first week of life due to auto diuresis. Infants should return to birth weight by 2 weeks of life.

Growth Velocity Goals:

Weight < 2000g	Weight > 2000g
•15-20 g/kg/day	•25-50 g/kg/day

[current weight (g) – prior weight (g)/# days/prior weight (kg)]

*Note: Steroids and diuretics can impair growth.

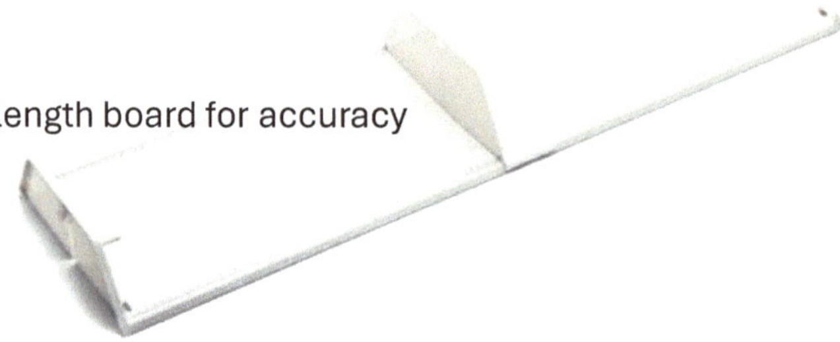

Length: 0.9 cm/week – should be measured using a length board for accuracy

HC: 0.9 cm/week preterm
0.5 cm/week term

Growth Goals

AAP

"approximate the rate of growth and composition of weight gain for a normal fetus of the same postmenstrual age while maintaining normal concentrations of nutrients in blood and other tissues"

ESPGHAN

"achieve growth similar to fetal growth coupled with satisfactory functional development"

- Preterm infants generally grow parallel to Fenton growth curve following initial physiological weight loss due to water balance changes.
- PNGF and EUGR definitions are based only on weight gain and do not consider linear growth, optimal body composition, or head growth as predictive of neurodevelopmental outcomes.
- Weight <10th percentile is NOT a stand-alone predictor of adverse neurodevelopmental outcomes.
- SGA babies are not expected to become AGA babies.
- Crossing percentile channels due to rapid weight gain risks overfeeding and does not promote optimal body composition.

Growth Curves

- The Fenton growth curve is used in preterm infants to 52 weeks of age.
- Weight, length, and head circumference are all on the same chart.

Defining Suboptimal Growth

Growth Velocity < goal

Birth Weight not regained by 2 weeks of life

Drop of > 2 channels on growth curve

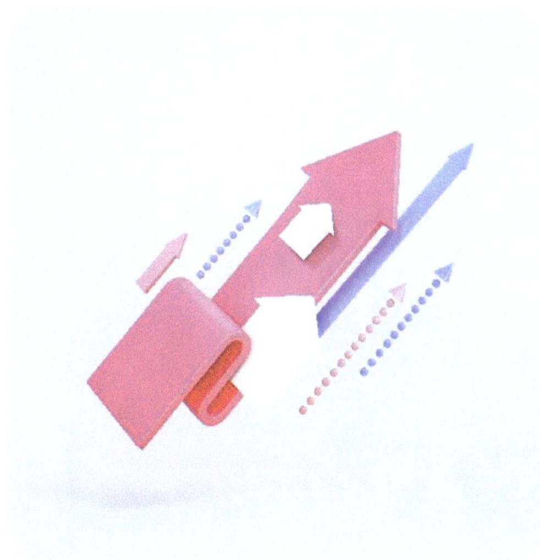

Z-Scores and Malnutrition

A z-score represents the standard deviation from 50th percentile.

Z-scores are calculated for weight-for-age, length-for-age, head circumference-for-age, and weight-for-length based on growth curve plot.

< -1.00 = mild malnutrition

< -2.00 = moderate malnutrition

< -3.00 = severe malnutrition

Term Growth Parameters: 25-50 g/day [current weight (g) – prior weight (g)/# days]

Interpretation of Sample Growth Curves

Example Below Curve, but Following Trajectory So Appropriate Growth

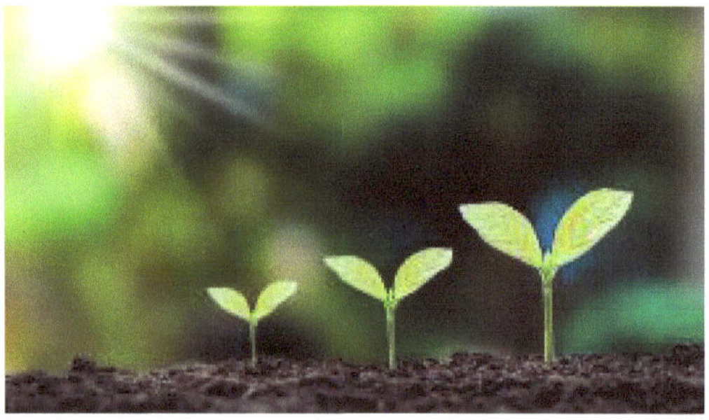

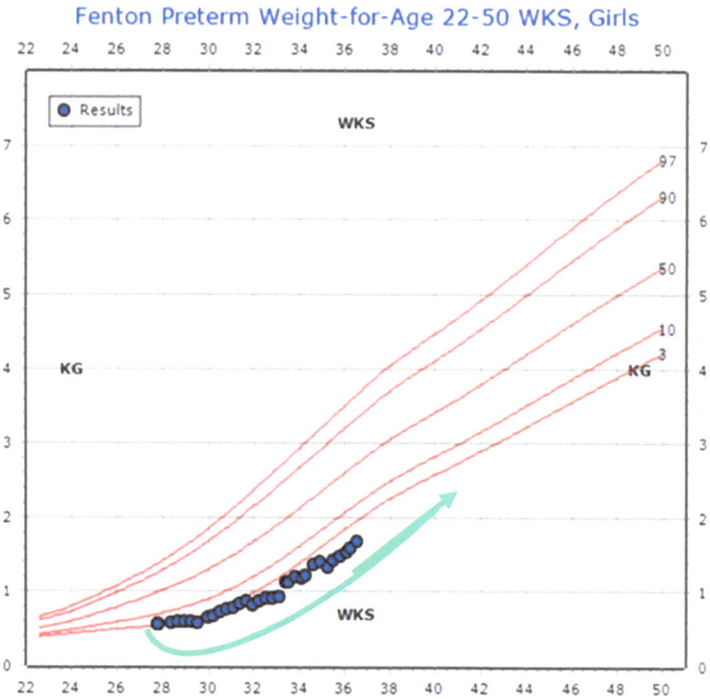

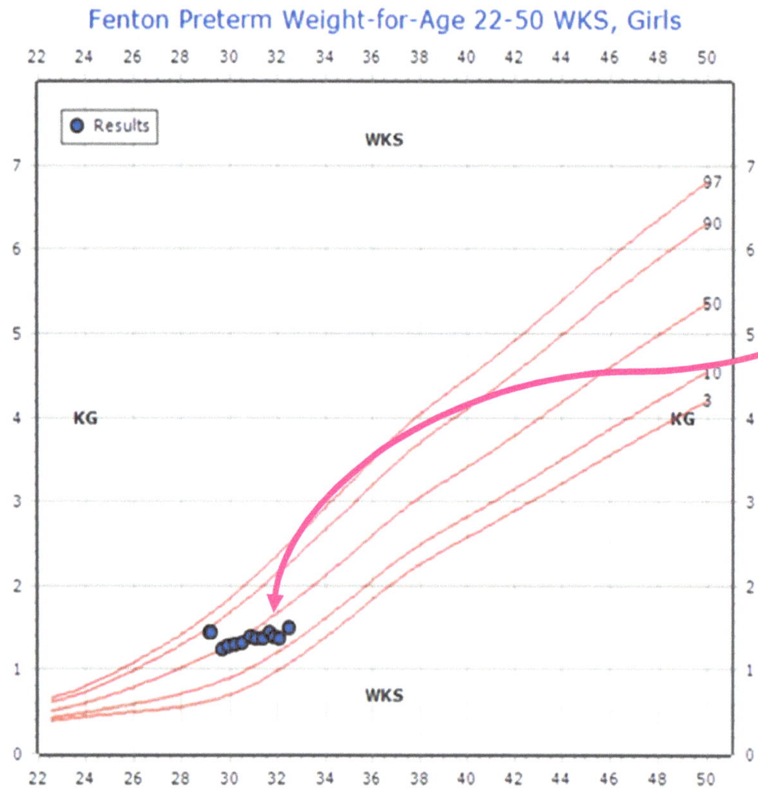

Example of Faltering Growth

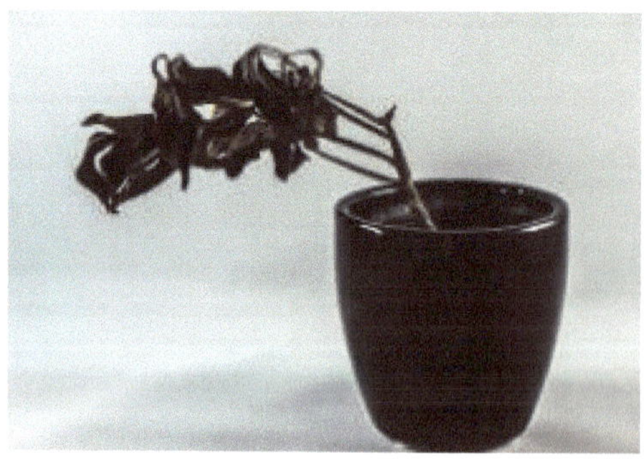

Strategies for Faltering Growth

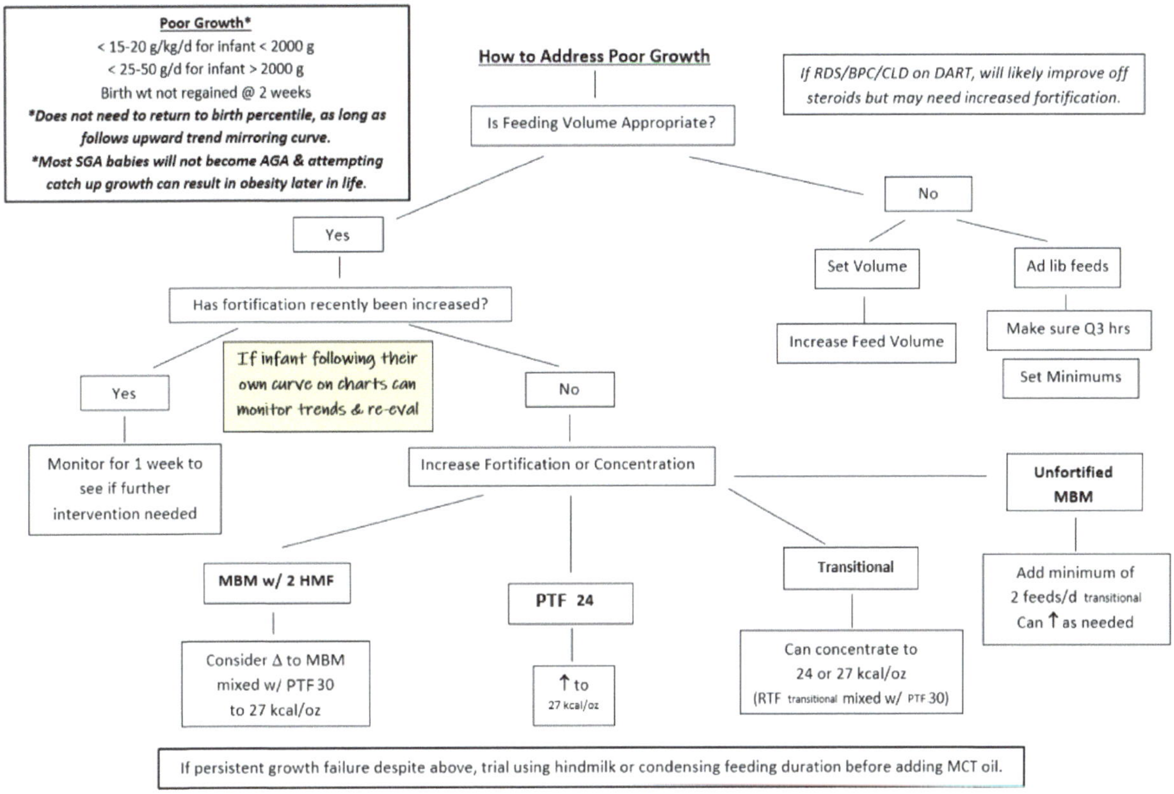

Additional Strategies

- Setting feeding minimum volumes
- Using hindmilk
- Adding formula to fortify MBM to exceed 24 kcal/oz.
- Concentrating formula

Use of MCT (medium-chain triglyceride) oils in addition to HM feeds can be associated with feeding intolerance and is not considered sterile, so it should not be recommended in practice.

What Is Hindmilk?

- Breast milk composition changes throughout the duration of the breastfeeding or pumping session.
- Foremilk is what the baby first accesses at the beginning of a feeding.
- Hindmilk is the milk produced towards the end of the feeding or expression.
  - When pumping, it often appears thick and creamy and is richer and more calorie dense than the foremilk.
  - It is more concentrated in fat to signal satiety at the end of a feeding.
  - Hindmilk can be useful in infants that are struggling to gain adequate weight with exclusive breast milk.
  - Consult Lactation for maternal support if hindmilk is needed.

See Appendices for Maternal Hindmilk Education.

Prefeeding Strategies

- SLP will get involved with micropreemies early in their NICU stay for prefeeding therapy.
- Oral stimulation can improve nutritive sucking and breastfeeding rates once infants are ready to start oral feeds. Often this is done with a pacifier, fingers, or mom's exposed nipple.
- Skin-to-skin care, once the infant is hemodynamically stable, can help regulate the sleep-wake cycle and maturation of the autonomic nervous system, which in turn can aid in feeding readiness.
- Infants need to learn to coordinate their suck, swallow, and breathe patterns.

Transition from EHMD

- Maternal breast milk fortified with Prolacta® should be transitioned to bovine-based fortifier when the infant weighs 1500 grams or is >34 weeks if SGA or history of NEC/feeding intolerance.
- Bovine HMF products are extensively hydrolyzed concentrated liquid formulations, which are designed to improve tolerance and decrease long-term risk of allergy.

Day	EHMD to MBM with HMF (bovine)	EHMD to Formula
1	2 parts MBM/PL to 1 part MBM w/ 1 HMF	2 parts BBM/PL to 1 part 24 cal preterm formula
2	1 part MBM/PL to 1 part MBM w/ 2 HMF	1 part BBM/PL to 1 part 24 cal preterm formula
3	MBM w/ 2 HMF	24 cal preterm formula (SSC24 or PE24)

Oral Issues Affecting Feeding

- SLP generally gets involved in feeding issues after 37 weeks CGA.

Ankyloglossia – Tongue-Tie

- Occurs when a short lingual frenulum or a tightly attached genioglossus muscle restricts tongue movement.
- Breastfeeding problems and/or poor latch can occur in some.
- No issues with bottle feeding are known.

Cleft Lip or Palate

- Cleft lip and cleft palate are openings or splits in the upper lip, roof of the mouth (palate), or both.
- Cleft lip and cleft palate result when facial structures that are developing in an unborn baby don't close completely.
- They can cause difficulty with feedings or difficulty swallowing, with potential for liquids or foods to come out through the nose.

Micrognathia

- Caused by impaired growth of the mandible, resulting in a smaller lower jaw.
- May cause upper respiratory obstruction in the neonate.
- Results in an oral cavity that is disproportionately small for the tongue.

Macroglossia

- Enlargement of the tongue, which can cause difficulties eating and swallowing.

Metabolic Bone Disease (MBD)/Osteopenia

- Preterm infants are at increased risk for Vitamin D deficiency and metabolic bone disease.
- Radiologic findings of Ricketts have been shown in 10-20% of ELBW infants despite nutritional interventions.

The recommended Vitamin D dosage is 400-1000 IU from reaching full EN through 6 months of age.

Risk due to prematurity, BW < 1500g, prolonged TPN > 1 month, prolonged steroid or diuretic use (>2 weeks)

↓

Labs present with ↑ALP > 600 and ↓Phos levels

↓

May see long-bone fractures on x-ray

↓

Nutrition Management: supplement additional 400 IU Vitamin D

Clinical Practice Guidelines for Metabolic Bone Disease

- Routine Screening should start at 1 month of life and should serum Alkaline phosphatase, phosphorus, and calcium.
- Infants should be receiving a baseline of 400 IU Vitamin D from PVS, bovine HMF, or preterm formula.
- For infants with ALP > 600 IU/L, supplement an additional Vitamin D 1 ml (400 IU) daily.
- For infants with Vitamin D deficiency, increase Vitamin D to 1.5 ml (600 IU) daily.

Normal Reference Values

ALP	< 600 IU/L
Serum Phosphorus	> 5.5 mg/dl
Serum Calcium iCa	8 – 10.5 mg/dl 1.2 -1.35 mmol/L *low calcium will be a late marker of bone mineral loss
25 OH-Vitamin D	>30 ng/ml * <20 ng/ml indicates deficiency
PTH	<100 pg/mL
Tubular Reabsorption of Phosphate (TRP)	85-95% **TRP = 1 – (Urine Phosphate/Urine Creatinine x Serum Creatinine/Serum Phosphate) x 100** *Use in evaluation of hypophosphatemia. Obtain Serum & urine studies around the same time. **TRP >95%** (ie. low urinary phosphate wasting) with low serum phosphorous suggests need for phosphate supplementation. Low TRP with high PTH suggests calcium deficiency.
Urine Ca/Creatinine Ratio	<3.8 mmol/mmol (1.3 mg/mg)
Xrays	Will not show signs of osteopenia until 30-40% bone mineral loss is present

Rustico, S. E., Calabria, A. C., & Garber, S. J. (2014). Metabolic bone disease of prematurity. Journal of clinical & translational endocrinology, 1(3), 85–91. https://doi.org/10.1016/j.jcte.2014.06.004

Nutrition Management of Specialty Populations

Respiratory Diseases

- Increased work of breathing causes high energy needs to support growth, and treatment with steroids impairs growth.
- Defined as chronic if continues to require positive pressure respiratory support or oxygen after 36 weeks CGA or 28 days of life.

AOP	BPD	CLD	CPIP
Apnea of Prematurity	Bronchopulmonary Dysplasia	Chronic Lung Disease	Chronic Pulmonary Insufficiency of Prematurity

Congenital Heart Disease (CHD)

- Birth defects that affect the heart structure and function affect systemic blood flow and increase baseline metabolic energy requirements.
- Infants with CHD may require surgery early in life and are at increased risk for malnutrition.

Most Common Types of CHD:

- Patent Ductus Arteriosus (PDA) – condition in which ductus fails to close after birth.
  - May require infant to be NPO for pharmacologic closure or ligation, which may need to be repeated.
  - Pharmacologic closure options: Indomethacin, Neoprofen, and Tylenol
- Atrial Septal Defect (ASD) – hole in heart wall between left and right atria
- Ventricular Septal Defect (VSD) – hole in heart wall between left and right ventricles
- Patent Foramen Ovale (PFO) – type of ASD
  - May close on its own.
  - Larger PFOs can increase risk of stroke and may need surgery to be closed.
- Pulmonary or Arterial Stenosis – narrowing of vessels impacting blood flow
- Tetralogy of Fallot – 4 heart defects, including pulmonary stenosis, VSD, overriding aorta, and right ventricular hypertrophy
- Transposition of Great Arteries (TGA) – aorta and pulmonary artery are switched from their normal positions in the heart
  - Life-threatening and requires surgery.
- Persistent Pulmonary Hypertension of the Newborn (PPHN) – high blood pressure in the lungs affecting oxygenation of the blood

Factors Impacting Nutrition

Increased metabolic demand	Heart failure may require fluid restrictions	Use of diuretics	Fatigue during feedings

ECMO – Extracorporeal Membrane Oxygenation

- Provides long-term machine support to heart and lungs.
- Energy needs are comparable to healthy infants, but protein needs are greater.
- ECMO increases protein catabolism due to stress and inflammation.
- A 7-day course of ECMO can result in up to 15% loss of lean body mass in neonates.

"Events" – Apnea and Bradycardia (A's & B's)

- Apnea is an irregular breathing pattern in which an infant stops breathing for > 15 seconds.
- Bradycardia is a slow heart rate, and it often follows apneic events in infants.
- These events are routinely monitored. Frequent events will delay progression to oral intake.

Neurologic Compromise

Intraventricular Hemorrhage (IVH)

- Bleeding in the brain that occurs within the first 4 days of life.
- Severe IVH may result in neurodevelopmental delays.

Hypoxemic Ischemic Encephalopathy (HIE)

- Brain damage caused by lack of oxygen to the brain either before or shortly after birth.
- May result in neurodevelopmental delays.

Body Cooling

- Goal is to slow energy expenditure to allow healing following moderate to severe HIE.
- Infants with moderate or severe HIE are cooled to a body temperature between 33.5°C-34.5°C within 6 h of birth.
- Infants continue cooling for 72 hours before being slowly rewarmed.
- Re-warming to a normal rectal temperature of 36.5-37°C occurs over at least 4 h at a rate of 0.5°C per hour.
- Enteral feeding should be withheld and PN provided until rewarming is complete.

GI Disorders and Alterations

Necrotizing Enterocolitis (NEC)

- Symptoms:

Emesis	Increased abdominal girth	Abdominal discoloration	Absence of stooling

- Requires NPO and TPN.
- Often appears on abdominal x-ray as pneumatosis.
- Risk peaks at 27-32 weeks CGA.
- EHMD can be protective, but use of hydrolyzed-protein fortifiers is generally safe.
- Early initiation of minimum enteral feeds does NOT increase the risk of NEC and showed benefits such as a shorter time to full enteral feeds, faster weight gain, improved feeding tolerance, decreased length of hospitalization, and reduced incidence of serious infections in VLBW infants.

Gastroschisis

- This rare birth defect occurs when the muscles and skin covering the abdomen do not fully develop before birth and the baby's intestines protrude through a hole in the abdominal wall near the umbilicus.
- This is life-threatening and requires surgery with bowel rest and TPN.

Omphalocele

- This rare birth defect occurs when the baby's abdominal organs, encased in a thin transparent membrane, protrude through a hole in the abdominal wall near the umbilicus.
- This is life-threatening and requires surgery with bowel rest and TPN.

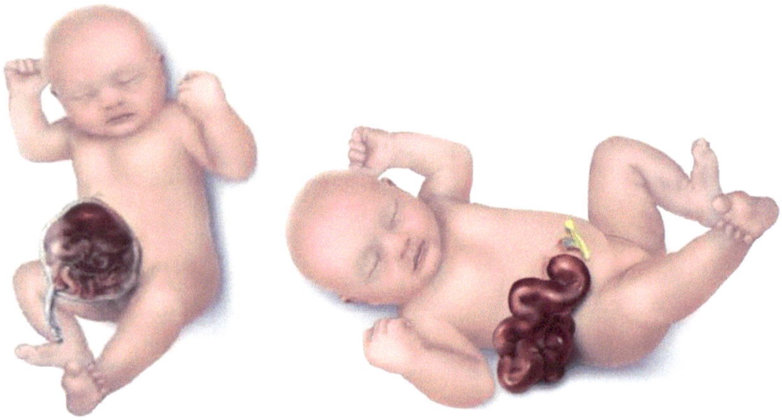

Omphalocele Gastroschisis

Image Citation: Verma, Richa. (2020). Congenital Anomalies of the Gastrointestinal Tract. 10.5772/intechopen.92588.

Gastroesophageal Reflux (GER)

- Defined as reflux of stomach contents into the esophagus, which typically improves with maturation and resolves by 1 year of age.
- The thickening of feeds in preterm infants has not been sufficiently studied to be considered safe and effective treatment.
- Use of commercial thickeners containing xanthan gum (Simply Thick) should be avoided due to the risk of NEC.
- Changing formulas is not recommended.

Biliary Atresia

- Presents with worsening jaundice unresponsive to phototherapy, elevated direct bilirubin and alkaline phosphatase (ALP) levels, cholestasis, dark urine, and gray stools.
- Causes biliary obstruction and requires timely surgery to prevent liver damage.

Neonatal Opiate Withdrawal Syndrome (NOWS)

- Previously known as NAS (Neonatal Abstinence Syndrome)
- Clinical Presentation:
  - Irritability
  - Increased muscle tone
  - Decreased sleep
  - Fevers
  - GI distress – vomiting or loose/watery stools
  - Feeding difficulties
- Eat, Sleep, Console (ESC) Screening
  - Evaluates the infant's ability to eat >1 oz or breastfeed well, sleep undisturbed > 1 hour, and be consoled.
- Treatment with medications in moderate to severe NOWS include morphine, buprenorphine (suboxone), phenobarbital.

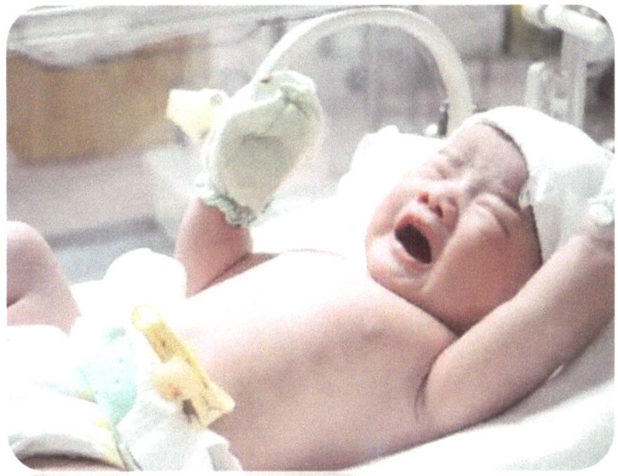

Nutrition Concerns in NOWS

Increased energy requirements due to tremors, tachypnea and poor sleep patterns

Frequent feeding difficulties, which can be associated with weight loss

- Most severe in initial phase of NOWS, usually 1-2 weeks
- Immature suck-swallow-breathe rhythms
- Prolonged sucking with fewer pauses, more spitting up and po refusal
- Unclear feeding cues

Loose stools common due to rapid gut transit time

- Opiate receptors in the GI tract become concentrated and are no longer stimulated.
- This is not necessarily a sign of intolerance and should not require formula change.

HM provision can decrease severity but maternal lactation rates are low.

NICU Graduation and Discharge Planning

- Use of a preterm discharge formula or a mixed diet of MBM and preterm discharge formula has been demonstrated to improve linear growth, lean body mass accretion, head circumference growth, and neurodevelopmental outcomes.
- ELBW infants may require continued feeding fortification or concentration post-discharge.
- Both Abbott and Mead Johnson offer discharge programs for NICU graduates.
    - As long as medically indicated, referral is compliant with Baby-Friendly© designation.
- Formula-fed infants should be transitioned to term formula once > 3600g.

Nutrition Planning for the NICU Graduate

NICU HEALTHCARE PROFESSIONAL: PROVIDE THIS FORM TO PEDIATRICIAN

Name:	**DOB:**	**Discharge Date:**

This infant is at nutrition risk, requiring as specialized nutrition plan due to (select all that apply):

- Prematurity (early or late preterm) ______ GA
- Very or extremely low birth wight ______ kg
- Intrauterine growth restriction
- Extrauterine growth restriction
- Suboptimal weight gain
- Low Phosphorus and/or high alkaline phosphatase
- Radiologic evidence of bone demineralization
- Volume Restriction
- Other: ______________________________

Discharge Feeding Plan & Recommendations

Method of Feeding (select all that apply):

Breast Bottle – Expressed BM Bottle – Formula Both Breast & Bottle Feeding tube

Human Milk w/ Fortification or Formula

Supplement Breastfeeding:

- BF alternating w/ expressed MBM + transitional powder 24 kcal/oz
  Recipe: 1 tsp formula per 90 ml MBM
- BF alternating w/ expressed MBM + transitional powder 27 kcal/oz
  Recipe: 1 tsp formula per 45 ml MBM

Expressed Maternal Breast Milk w/ Fortification:

- Expressed MBM + Human Milk Fortifier
  (not to exceed 22 packets/day)
    - 1 pack HMF per 50 ml MBM
    - 2 packs HMF per 50 ml MBM
    - Feeding Volume______ ml MBM + ____ packets HMF
- Expressed MBM + Transitional Preterm Formula
    - 24 kcal/oz = 90 ml MBM + 1 tsp formula powder
    - Feeding Volume ______ ml MBM +____ tsp formula powder
    - 27 kcal/oz = 45 ml MBM + 1 tsp formula powder
    - Feeding Volume ______ ml MBM +____ tsp formula powder

Formula ☐ Exclusive ☐ If MBM unavailable

Transitional Preterm Formula:
(EnfaCare or Neosure)

- Ready to feed (22 kcal/oz)
- Powder, per mixing instructions, below:
    - 22 kcal/oz (2 fl oz water + 1 scoop)
    - 24 kcal/oz (5 ½ fl oz water + 3 scoops)
    - 27 kcal/oz (8 fl oz water + 5 scoops)
    - 30 kcal/oz (7 fl oz water + 5 scoops)
    - All Feeds
    - Every Other Feed

Current Feeding Volume: ________ ml/day

Vitamins: Poly-Vi-Sol w/ Iron 0.5 ml/day Poly-Vi-Sol w/ Iron 1 ml/day Vitamin D 400 IU *(1 ml)/day* None

Recommendations:

The following fortification timeline is based on infant birth weight:

Birth Weight	**Supplement Duration**
<750 grams	Up to 12 months postnatal
751 – 1000 grams	Up to 9 months postnatal
1001 – 1500 grams	Up to 6 months postnatal
1501 – 1800 grams	Up to 3 months postnatal

****Please check Ca, Phos & ALP at 4 weeks post-discharge.*

If maternal milk supply decreases & more formula is needed, a dietitian consult may be needed.

If growth becomes excessive, can drop to 22 kcal/oz.

HMF should be discontinued once infant reaches 3.5 kg. At this point, change to 22 cal transitional formula every other feed.

______________________________ ______________

Signature of NICU Healthcare Professional (Physician, NNP, RD, RN) **Date/Time:**

Telephone:	Email:

References

1. Koletzko B, Cheah FC, Domellöf M, Poindexter BB, Vain N, van Goudoever JB (eds): Nutritional Care of Preterm Infants, 2nd Ed, Karger, 2021.
2. Pediatric Nutrition Reference Guide, 11th Edition, Texas Children's Hospital, 2016.
3. Baby-Friendly USA ~ Upholding the Highest Standards of Infant Feeding Care (babyfriendlyusa.org).
4. Ehrenkranz RA, Dusick AM, Vohr BR, et al. Growth in the Neonatal Intensive Care Unit Influences Neurodevelopmental and Growth Outcomes of Extremely Low Birth Weight Infants. Pediatrics 2006; 117 (4): 1253-1261. DOI: 10.1542/peds.2005-1368.
5. Arslanoglu S, Boquien CY, King C, Lamireau D, Tonetto P, Barnett D, et al. Fortification of Human Milk for Preterm Infants: Update and Recommendations of the European Milk Bank Association (EMBA) Working Group on Human Milk Fortification. Front Pediatr. 2019;7:76.
6. Banait N, Basu S, Desai P, et al. Feeding of Low Birth Weight Neonates. Journal of Neonatology. 2020;34(1-2):28-51. https://doi.org/10.1177%2F0973217920938522.
7. Bergner, Erynn M et al. "Human Milk Fortification: A Practical Analysis of Current Evidence." Clinics in perinatology vol. 49,2 (2022): 447-460. doi:10.1016/j.clp.2022.02.010.
8. Thoene M, Anderson-Berry A. A review of best evidenced-based enteral and parenteral nutrition support practices for preterm infants born <1,500 grams. Pediatr Med 2018; 1:6. http://dx.doi.org/10.21037/pm.2.
9. Hair AB, Hawthorne KM, Chetta KE, Abrams SA. Human milk feeding supports adequate growth in infants < 1250 grams birth weight. BMC Research Notes, 2013, 6:459. http://www.biomedcentral.com/1756-0500/6/459.
10. Huston R, et al. Early fortification of enteral feedings for infants <1250 grams birth weight receiving a human milk diet including human milk-based fortifier. J Neonatal Perinatal Med. 2020;13(2):215-221. https://pubmed.ncbi.nlm.nih.gov/31707377.
11. Markell, A. Nutrition guidelines for an exclusive human milk diet. Neonatal Intensive Care, 2016; 29: 18.
12. Section on Breastfeeding, Eidelman AI et al. Breastfeeding and the Use of Human Milk. Pediatrics March 2012; 129 (3): e827–e841. https://doi.org/10.1542/peds.2011-3552.
13. Banait N, Basu S, Desai P, et al. Feeding of Low Birth Weight Neonates. Journal of Neonatology. 2020;34(1-2):28-51. https://doi.org/10.1177%2F0973217920938522.
14. Hay WW. Nutritional Support Strategies for the Preterm Infant in the Neonatal Intensive Care Unit. Pediatri Gastroenterol Heaptol Nutr 2018; 21 (4): 234-247. https://doi.org/10.5223/pghn.2018.21.4.234.
15. Thoene M, Anderson-Berry A. Early Enteral Feeding in Preterm Infants: A Narrative Review of the Nutritional, Metabolic, and Developmental Benefits. Nutrients. 2021 Jul 1;13(7):2289. https://doi.org/10.3390%2Fnu13072289.
16. Kwok TC, Dorling J, Gale C. Early enteral feeding in preterm infants. Semin Perinatol. 2019;43(7):151159. https://doi.org/10.1053/j.semperi.2019.06.007.
17. Hair et al. Randomized trial of human milk cream as a supplement to standard fortification of an exclusive human milk-based diet in infants 750-1250 g birth weight. The Journal of Pediatrics, 2014. https://doi.org/10.1016/j.jpeds.2014.07.005.
18. Rochow N, Fusch G, Ali A, et al. Individualized target fortification of breast milk with protein, carbohydrates, and fat for preterm infants: A double-blind randomized controlled trial. Clinical Nutrition 2021; 40: 54-63. https://doi.org/10.1016/j.clnu.2020.04.031.
19. Morlacchi L, Mallardi D, Gianni ML, et al. Is targeted fortification of human breast milk an optimal nutrition strategy for preterm infants? An interventional study. J Transl Med 2016; 14: 195-202. DOI: 10.1186/s12967-016-0957-y.
20. Parat S, Raza P, Kamleh M, et al. Targeted Breast Milk Fortification for Very Low Birth Weight (VLBW) Infants: Nutritional Intake, Growth Outcome and Body Composition. Nutrients 2020; 12: 1156-1166. DOI: 10.3390/nu12041156.
21. Fabrizio V, Trzaski JM, Brownell EA, et al. Individualized versus standard diet fortification for growth and development in preterm infants receiving human milk. Cochrane Database Syst Rev. 2020;11(11):CD013465. Published 2020 Nov 23. doi:10.1002/14651858.CD013465.pub2.
22. Seliga-Siwecka, J., Chmielewska, A. & Jasińska, K. Effect of targeted vs standard fortification of breast milk on growth and development of preterm infants (≤ 32 weeks): study protocol for a randomized controlled trial. Trials 21, 946 (2020). https://doi.org/10.1186/s13063-020-04841-x.
23. Abiramalatha T, Thanigainathan S, Ninan B. Routine monitoring of gastric residual for prevention of necrotising enterocolitis in preterm infants. Cochrane Database Syst Rev. 2019 Jul 9;7(7):CD012937. https://doi.org/10.1002%2F14651858.CD012937.pub2.
24. Elia, S., Ciarcià, M., Miselli, F. et al. Effect of selective gastric residual monitoring on enteral intake in preterm infants. Ital J Pediatr 48, 30 (2022). https://doi.org/10.1186/s13052-022-01208-7

25. Isemann B, Mueller EW, Narendran V and Akinbi H. Impact of Early Sodium Supplementation on Hyponatremia and Growth in Premature Infants: A Randomized Controlled Trial. J Parenter Enteral Nutr, 2016; 40 (3): 342-349.
26. Bischoff AR, Tomlinson C and Belik J. Sodium Intake Requirements for Preterm Neonates: Review and Recommendations. JPGN 2016; 63: e123-e129.
27. Segar DE, Segar EK, Harshman LA, et al. Physiological Approach to Sodium Supplementation in Preterm Infants. Am J Perinatol 2018; 35: 994-1000.
28. Shaikhkhalil AK, Curtiss J, Puthoff TD and Valentine CJ. Enteral Zinc Supplementation and Growth in Extremely-Low-Birth-Weight Infants With Chronic Lung Disease. JPGN 2014; 58: 183-187. DOI: 10.1097/MPG.0000000000000145.
29. Terin G, Canani RB, Di Chiara M, et al. Zinc in Early Life: A Key Element in the Fetus and Preterm Neonate. Nutrients 2015; 7:10427-10446. DOI: 10.3390/nu7125542.
30. Fenton TR, Anderson D, Groh-Wargo S et al. An Attempt to Standardize the Calculation of Growth Velocity of Preterm Infants — Evaluation of Practical Bedside Methods. J Pediatr 2018; 196: 77-83. https://doi.org10.1016/j.jpeds.2017.10.005.
31. Growth Charts - WHO Child Growth Standards (cdc.gov).
32. Vander Veer, R. Establishing a Zinc Supplementation Protocol for Growth Failure in the Neonatal Intensive Care Unit. PNPG Building Block for Life 2019; 43: 1-7.
33. Robinson DT, Calkins KL, Chen Y, et al. Guidelines for parenteral nutrition in preterm infants: the American Society for Parenteral and Enteral Nutrition. J Parenter Enteral Nutr. 2023;47:830-858. doi:10.1002/jpen.2550
34. Wang N, Zhang J, Wang B, Yu Z, et al. Transition From Parenteral to Enteral Nutrition and Postnatal Growth in Very Preterm Infants During Their First 28 Days of Life. Frontiers in Pediatrics 2022; 10: 775667. https://doi.org/10.3389/fped.2022.775667.
35. Liotto N, Amato O, Piemontese P, Menis C, Orsi A, Corti MG, Colnaghi M, Cecchetti V, Pugni L, Mosca F, Roggero P. Protein Intakes during Weaning from Parenteral Nutrition Drive Growth Gain and Body Composition in Very Low Birth Weight Preterm Infants. Nutrients. 2020 May 2;12(5):1298. https://doi.org/10.3390%2Fnu12051298.
36. Fenton, T.R., Cormack, B., Goldberg, D. et al. "Extrauterine growth restriction" and "postnatal growth failure" are misnomers for preterm infants. J Perinatol 40, 704–714 (2020). https://doi.org/10.1038/s41372-020-0658-5.
37. Lubbe W. (2018). Clinicians guide for cue-based transition to oral feeding in preterm infants: An easy-to-use clinical guide. Journal of evaluation in clinical practice, 24(1), 80–88. https://doi.org/10.1111/jep.12721.
38. Rustico, S. E., Calabria, A. C., & Garber, S. J. (2014). Metabolic bone disease of prematurity. Journal of clinical & translational endocrinology, 1(3), 85–91. https://doi.org/10.1016/j.jcte.2014.06.004.
39. Common conditions treated in the NICU | March of Dimes.
40. Mosalli R. (2012). Whole body cooling for infants with hypoxic-ischemic encephalopathy. Journal of clinical neonatology, 1(2), 101–106. https://doi.org/10.4103/2249-4847.96777.
41. Verma R (2021) Congenital Anomalies of the Gastrointestinal Tract. Congenital Anomalies in Newborn Infants - Clinical and Etiopathological Perspectives. IntechOpen. Available at: http://dx.doi.org/10.5772/intechopen.92588.
42. Martin R and Hibb AM. Gastroesophageal reflux in premature infants. Up To Date. Gastroesophageal reflux in premature infants - UpToDate. Accessed 7/2/24.
43. Patrick SW, Barfield WD, Poindexter BB, AAP COMMITTEE ON FETUS AND NEWBORN, COMMITTEE ON SUBSTANCE USE AND PREVENTION. Neonatal Opioid Withdrawal Syndrome. Pediatrics. 2020;146(5):e2020029074.
44. Verma, Richa. (2020). Congenital Anomalies of the Gastrointestinal Tract. 10.5772/intechopen.92588.

APPENDICES

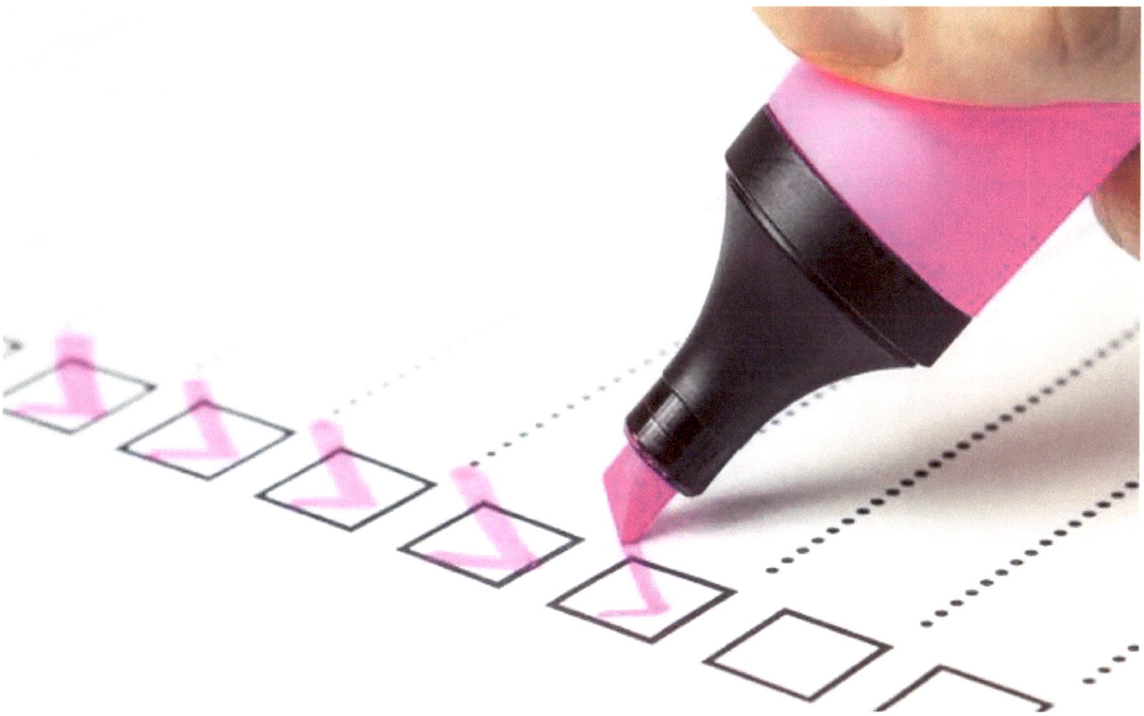

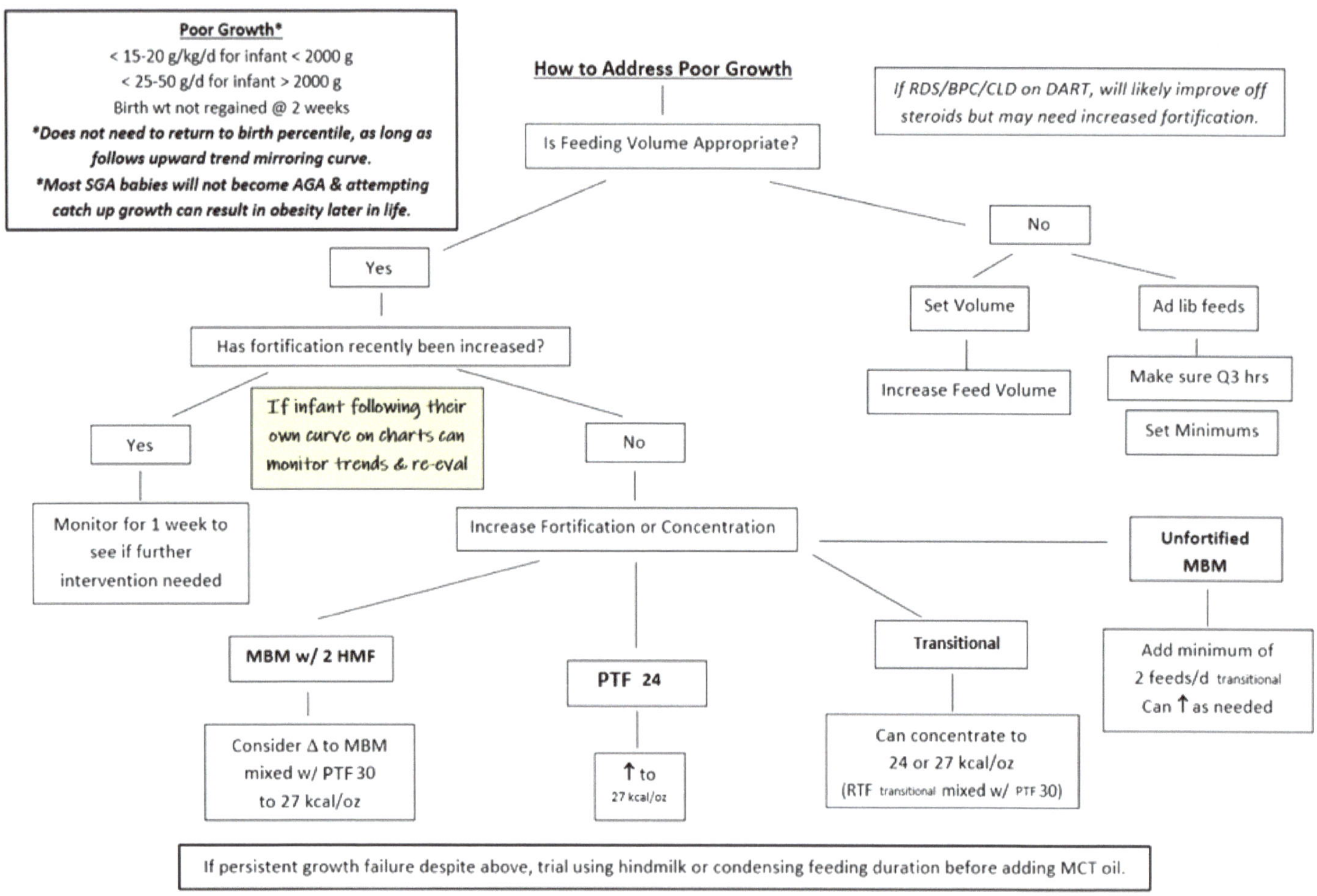
Poor Growth*
< 15-20 g/kg/d for infant < 2000 g
< 25-50 g/d for infant > 2000 g
Birth wt not regained @ 2 weeks
*Does not need to return to birth percentile, as long as follows upward trend mirroring curve.
*Most SGA babies will not become AGA & attempting catch up growth can result in obesity later in life.
How to Address Poor Growth
If RDS/BPC/CLD on DART, will likely improve off steroids but may need increased fortification.
Is Feeding Volume Appropriate?
Yes
No
Set Volume
Ad lib feeds
Increase Feed Volume
Make sure Q3 hrs
Set Minimums
Has fortification recently been increased?
Yes
If infant following their own curve on charts can monitor trends & re-eval
No
Monitor for 1 week to see if further intervention needed
Increase Fortification or Concentration
Unfortified MBM
Add minimum of 2 feeds/d transitional Can ↑ as needed
MBM w/ 2 HMF
PTF 24
Transitional
Consider Δ to MBM mixed w/ PTF 30 to 27 kcal/oz
↑ to 27 kcal/oz
Can concentrate to 24 or 27 kcal/oz (RTF transitional mixed w/ PTF 30)
If persistent growth failure despite above, trial using hindmilk or condensing feeding duration before adding MCT oil.

Fetal-Infant Growth Chart for Preterm Infants

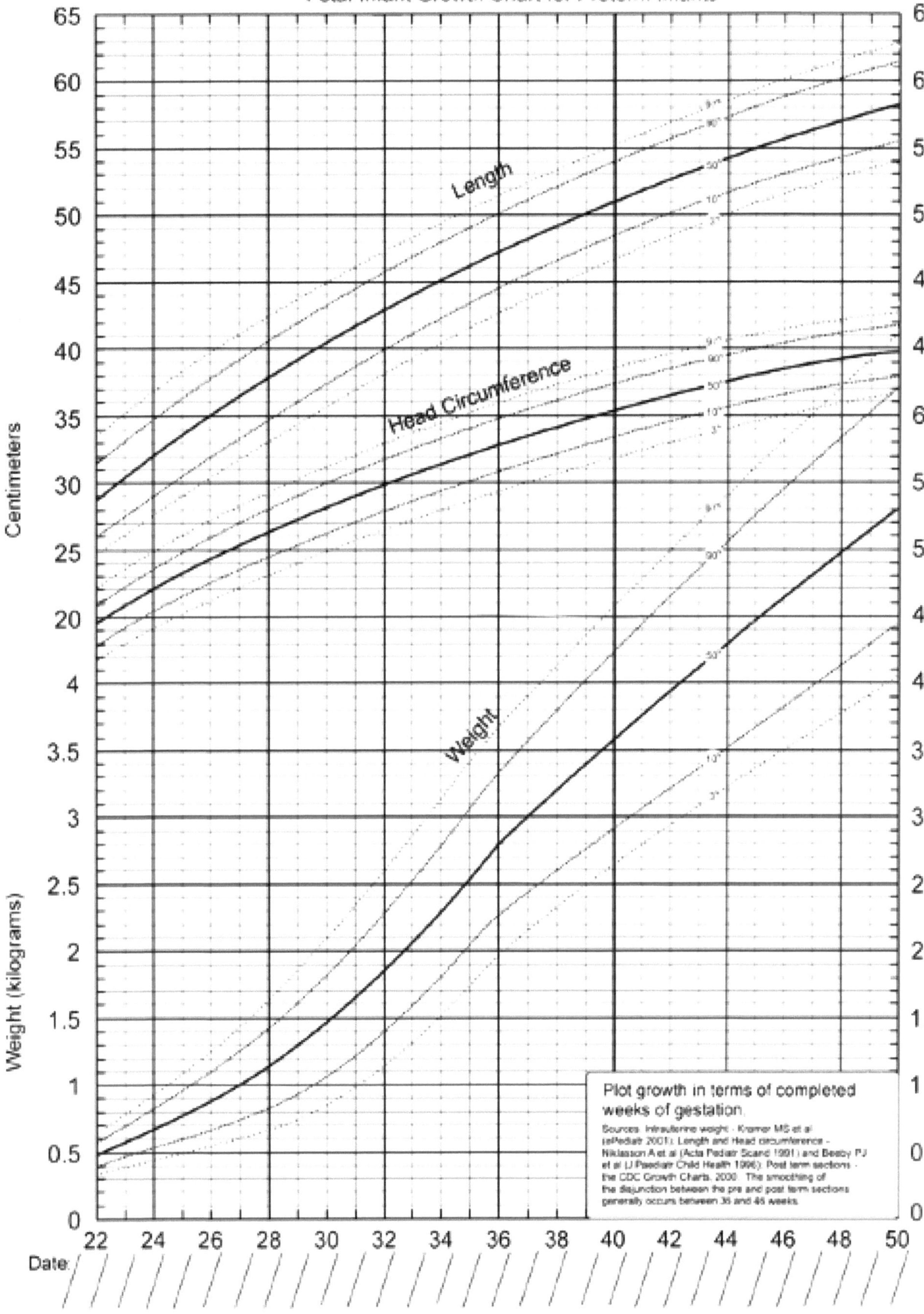

Citation: Fenton TR. BMC Pediatr. 2003 Dec 16; 3(1): 13

Birth to 24 months: Boys
Head circumference-for-age and Weight-for-length percentiles

NAME ____________________

RECORD # __________

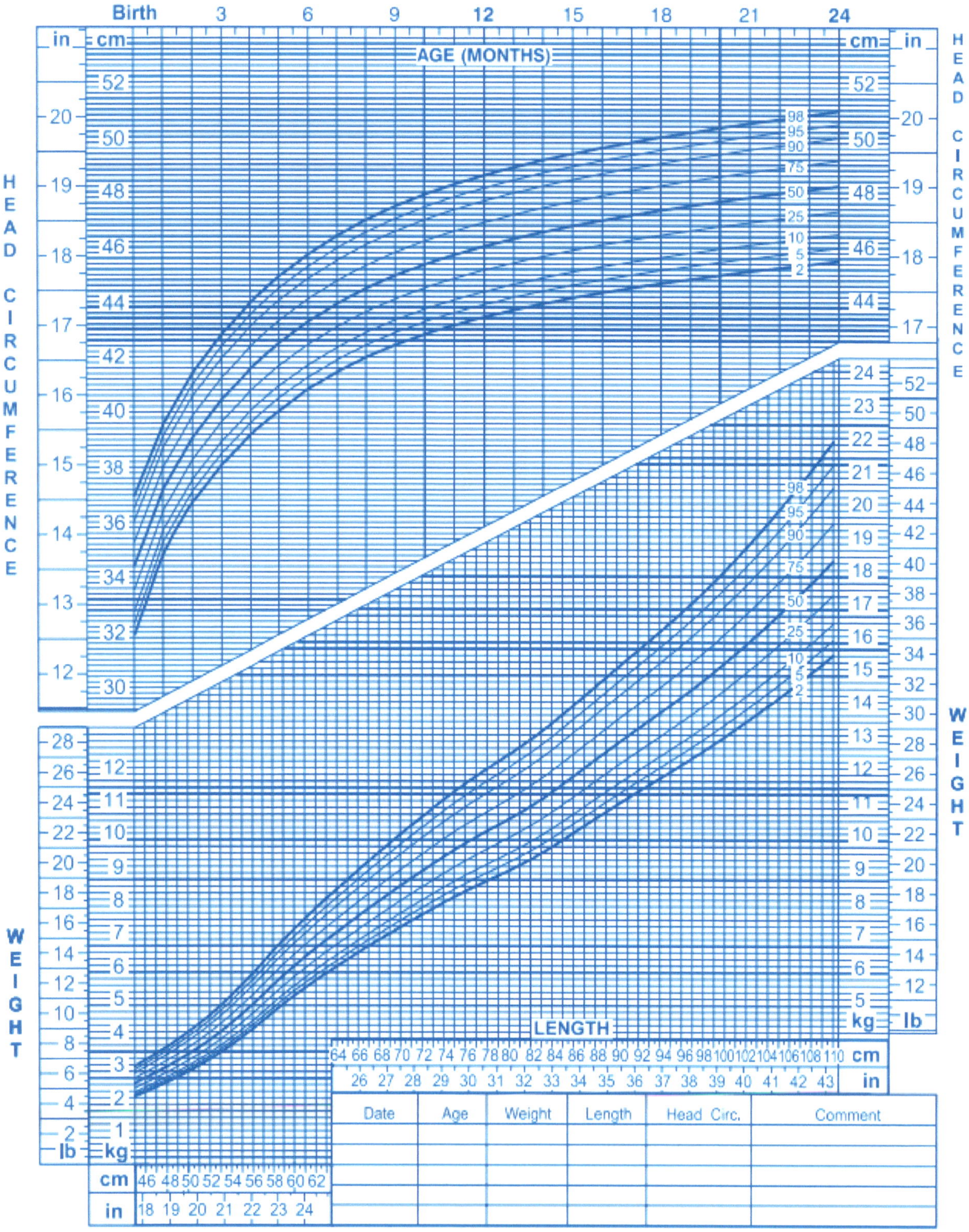

Date	Age	Weight	Length	Head Circ.	Comment

Published by the Centers for Disease Control and Prevention, November 1, 2009
SOURCE: WHO Child Growth Standards (http://www.who.int/childgrowth/en)

CDC

Birth to 24 months: Boys
Length-for-age and Weight-for-age percentiles

NAME ____________________

RECORD # ____________

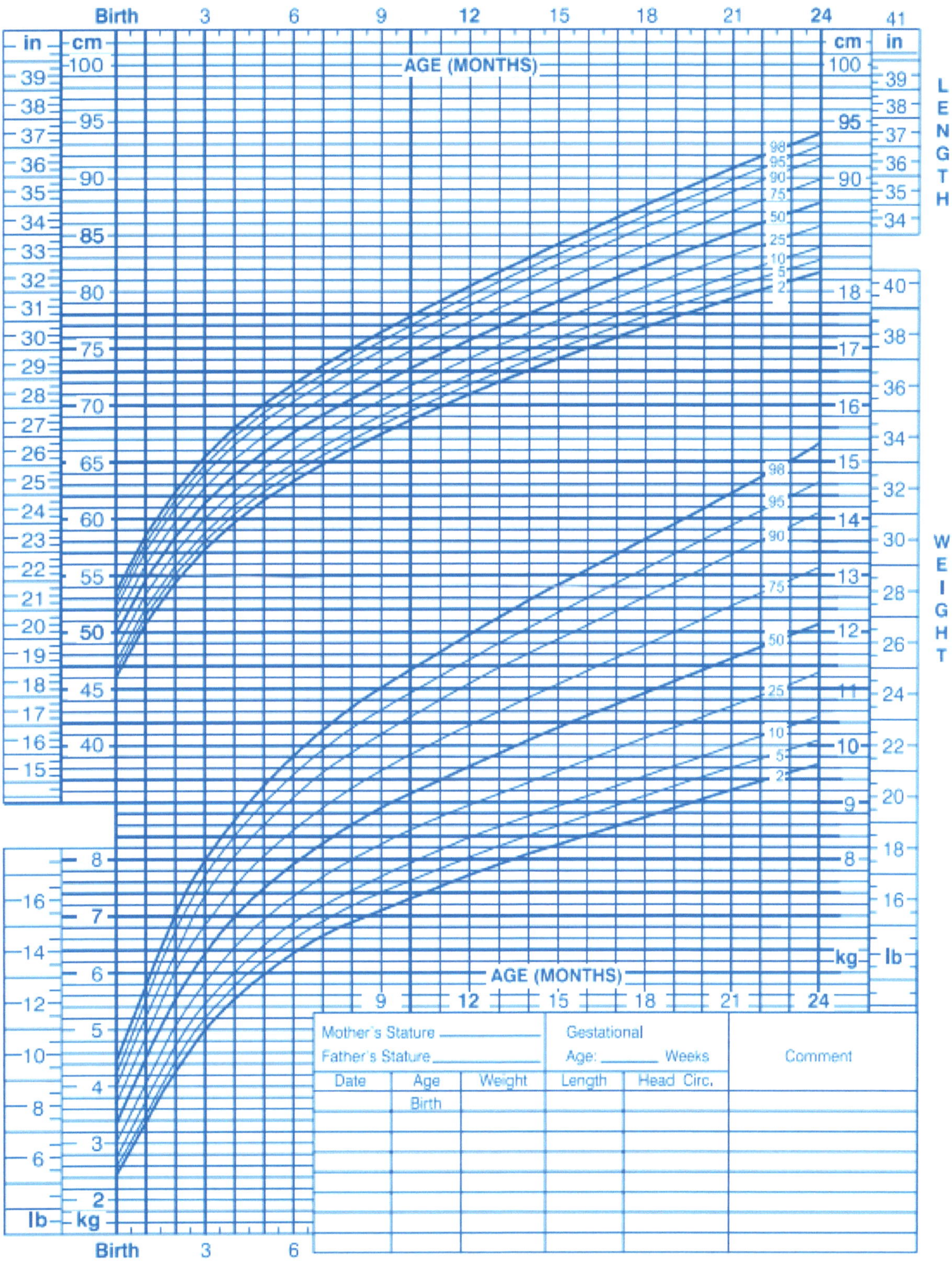

Mother's Stature ______			Gestational Age: ______ Weeks		Comment
Father's Stature ______					
Date	Age	Weight	Length	Head Circ.	
	Birth				

Published by the Centers for Disease Control and Prevention, November 1, 2009
SOURCE: WHO Child Growth Standards (http://www.who.int/childgrowth/en)

SAFER · HEALTHIER · PEOPLE™

Birth to 24 months: Girls
Head circumference-for-age and Weight-for-length percentiles

NAME ______________________

RECORD # __________

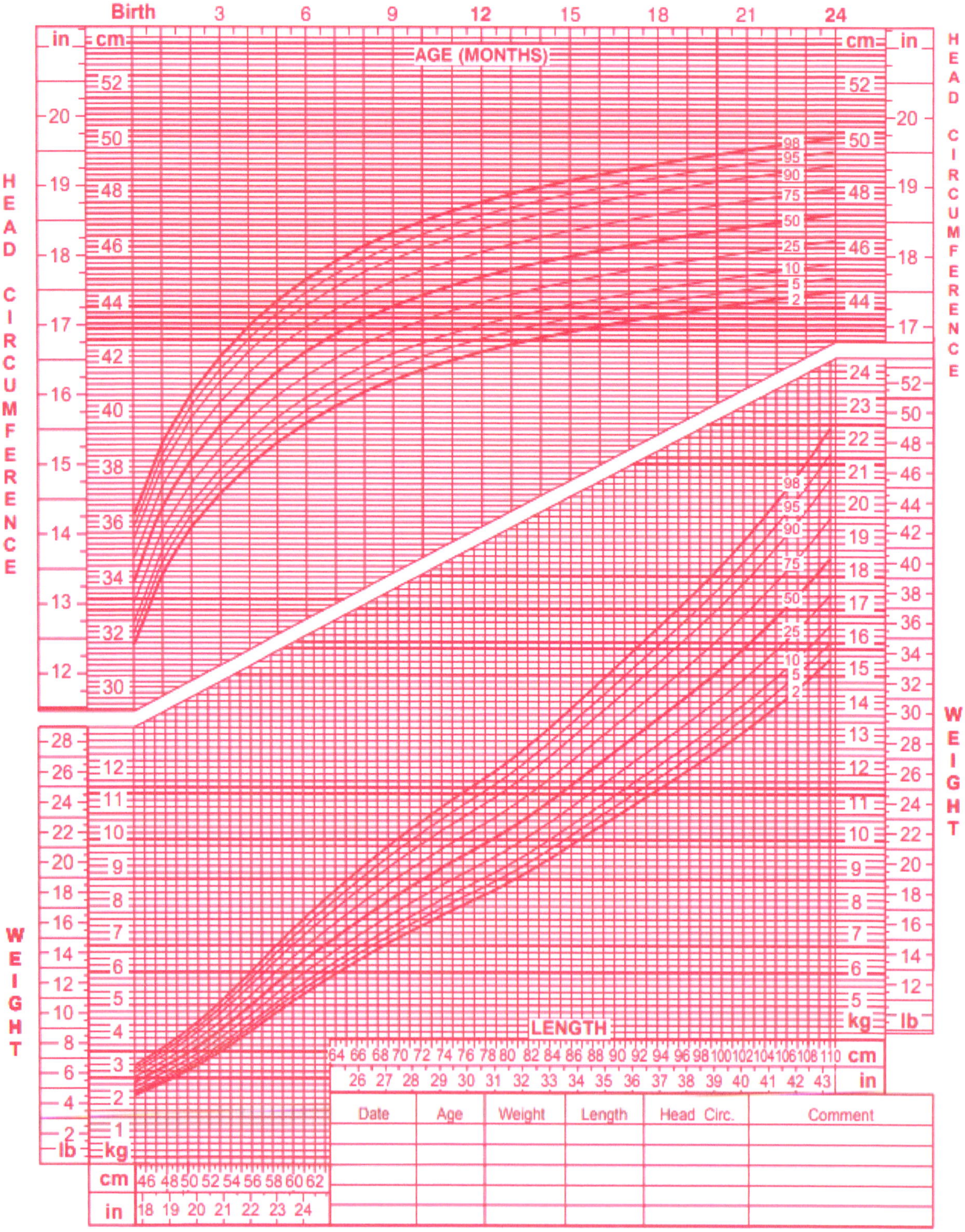

Date	Age	Weight	Length	Head Circ.	Comment

Published by the Centers for Disease Control and Prevention, November 1, 2009
SOURCE: WHO Child Growth Standards (http://www.who.int/childgrowth/en)

Birth to 24 months: Girls
Length-for-age and Weight-for-age percentiles

NAME ______________________

RECORD # __________

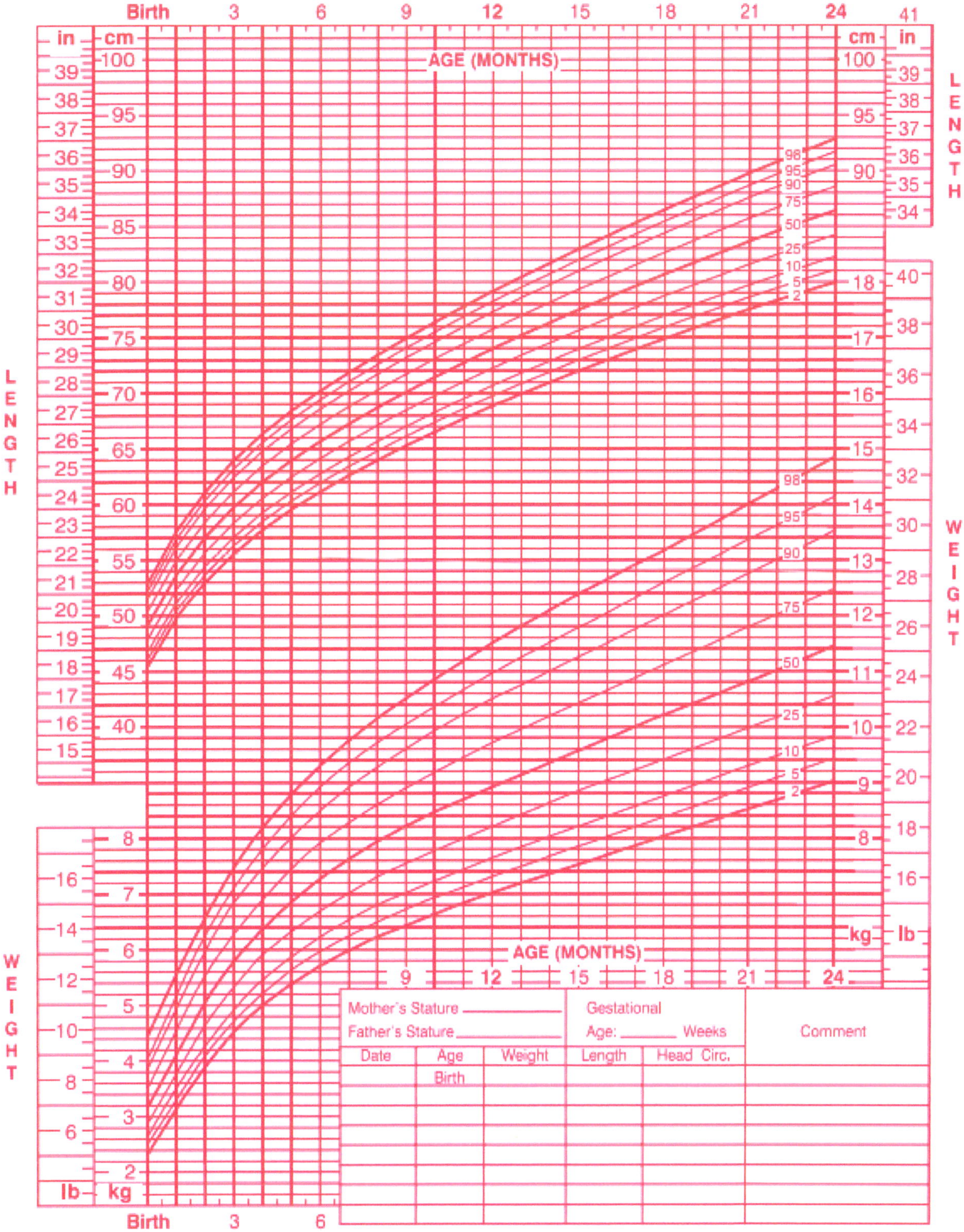

Mother's Stature ______________ Father's Stature ______________

Gestational Age: ________ Weeks

Date	Age	Weight	Length	Head Circ.	Comment
	Birth				

Published by the Centers for Disease Control and Prevention, November 1, 2009
SOURCE: WHO Child Growth Standards (http://www.who.int/childgrowth/en)

Nutrition Planning for the NICU Graduate

NICU HEALTHCARE PROFESSIONAL: PROVIDE THIS FORM TO PEDIATRICIAN

Name:	**DOB:**	**Discharge Date:**

This infant is at nutrition risk, requiring as specialized nutrition plan due to (select all that apply):

- Prematurity (early or late preterm) ______ GA
- Very or extremely low birth wight _______ kg
- Intrauterine growth restriction
- Extrauterine growth restriction
- Suboptimal weight gain
- Low Phosphorus and/or high alkaline phosphatase
- Radiologic evidence of bone demineralization
- Volume Restriction
- Other: ________________________________

Discharge Feeding Plan & Recommendations

Method of Feeding (select all that apply):

Breast | Bottle – Expressed BM | Bottle – Formula | Both Breast & Bottle | Feeding tube

Human Milk w/ Fortification or Formula

Supplement Breastfeeding:

- BF alternating w/ expressed MBM + transitional powder 24 kcal/oz
  Recipe: 1 tsp formula per 90 ml MBM
- BF alternating w/ expressed MBM + transitional powder 27 kcal/oz
  Recipe: 1 tsp formula per 45 ml MBM

Expressed Maternal Breast Milk w/ Fortification:

- Expressed MBM + Human Milk Fortifier
  (not to exceed 22 packets/day)
  - 1 pack HMF per 50 ml MBM
  - 2 packs HMF per 50 ml MBM
  - Feeding Volume_____ ml MBM + ____ packets HMF
- Expressed MBM + Transitional Preterm Formula
  - 24 kcal/oz = 90 ml MBM + 1 tsp formula powder
  - Feeding Volume _____ ml MBM +____ tsp formula powder
  - 27 kcal/oz = 45 ml MBM + 1 tsp formula powder
  - Feeding Volume _____ ml MBM +____ tsp formula powder

Formula

☐ Exclusive ☐ If MBM unavailable

Transitional Preterm Formula:
(EnfoCare or Neosure)

- Ready to feed (22 kcal/oz)
- Powder, per mixing instructions, below:
  - 22 kcal/oz (2 fl oz water + 1 scoop)
  - 24 kcal/oz (5 ½ fl oz water + 3 scoops)
  - 27 kcal/oz (8 fl oz water + 5 scoops)
  - 30 kcal/oz (7 fl oz water + 5 scoops)
  - All Feeds
  - Every Other Feed

Current Feeding Volume: ________ ml/day

Vitamins: Poly-Vi-Sol w/ Iron 0.5 ml/day | Poly-Vi-Sol w/ Iron 1 ml/day | Vitamin D 400 IU *(1 ml)*/day | None

Recommendations:

The following fortification timeline is based on infant birth weight:

Birth Weight	Supplement Duration
<750 grams	Up to 12 months postnatal
751 – 1000 grams	Up to 9 months postnatal
1001 – 1500 grams	Up to 6 months postnatal
1501 – 1800 grams	Up to 3 months postnatal

****Please check Ca, Phos & ALP at 4 weeks post-discharge.*

If maternal milk supply decreases & more formula is needed, a dietitian consult may be needed.
If growth becomes excessive, can drop to 22 kcal/oz.

HMF should be discontinued once infant reaches 3.5 kg. At this point, change to 22 cal transitional formula every other feed.

____ ______________
Signature of NICU Healthcare Professional (Physician, NNP, RD, RN) **Date/Time:**

Telephone:	Email:

Learning about Hindmilk and your Baby's Growth

Breast milk changes during breastfeeding or pumping sessions.

Foremilk is what your baby gets at the beginning of a feeding or pumping session.

Hindmilk is the what your baby gets towards the end of the feeding or pumping session.

What is Hindmilk?

Hindmilk looks thick and creamy and has more calories than foremilk. This is because it has the fat that tells your baby they are full at the end of a feeding. Hindmilk can help babies that do not gain enough weight with only breast milk.

The foods you eat will not change the amount of fat in your milk, but you can increase the amount of fat and calories in your milk by changing the way you pump. This is done by separating your milk.

To do this, you will need to make more milk than your baby eats every day. If you know how much you usually get from each pumping session, you can measure out and remove the first 1/3 that you pump (your foremilk). For example, if you usually pump 60 ml on each breast, then you will remove the first 20 ml of milk from each breast. **Ask a member of your care team for help if you are unsure or need help measuring what 1/3 of a pumping session is for you.**

After you finish pumping, you will use the leftover milk (your hindmilk) from the end of your pumping session to feed your baby. Your baby will still need the same total amount of milk as before for each feeding. That is why you'll need to make more milk than your baby eats.

A Lactation Consultant can help teach you how to pump and separate out your hindmilk.

Expressing Hindmilk

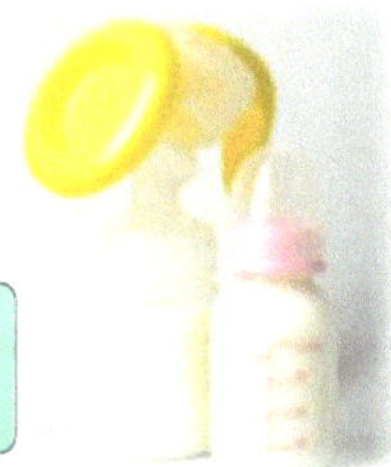

Make sure you wash your hands before pumping and separating your milk.

Have extra breast milk storage containers ready.

When you start pumping your breast milk, it will be thin and watery. Pump for about 2 minutes, then remove the collection container from the pump. This will contain foremilk. Label and freeze this and save it until your baby gets older and starts to wean off breast milk.

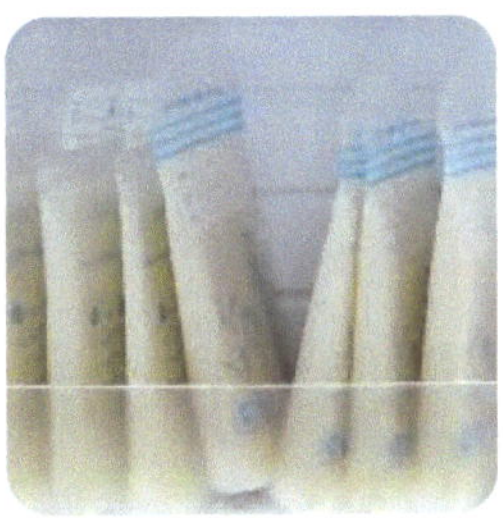

Then, place a new collection container on your breast pump and continue pumping until your breast is empty. This thicker, creamier breast milk that you get at the end of your pumping session is your hindmilk.

It can be helpful to massage your breasts while you pump because this helps add more fat to your milk.

If you are directly breastfeeding, you can pump for 2 minutes to remove the foremilk before putting your baby to your breast.

Nutrition for Breastfeeding Moms

Human breast milk is the best nutrition source for your baby. It has a balance of carbohydrates, protein, fat, water and other nutrients that are easily digested and absorbed, and its composition naturally changes as your baby's needs change. It also has protective factors against infection and allergies.

Breastfeeding requires more calories, protein, vitamins and minerals than you needed before pregnancy. Calorie needs can increase by up to 400 calories per day.

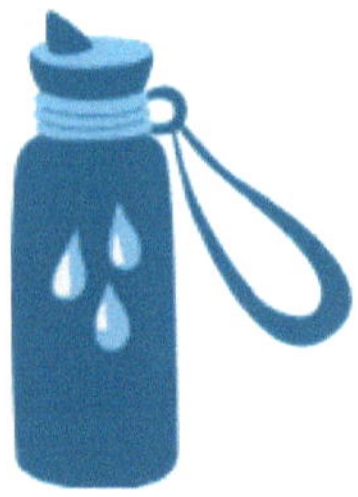

Stay Hydrated

- Hydration is the most important factor that can help improve your breast milk production volumes.
- Drink 12 (8 oz) caffeine-free beverages per day.
- Keep fluids readily available and drink a beverage each time you breastfeed your baby.

Diet

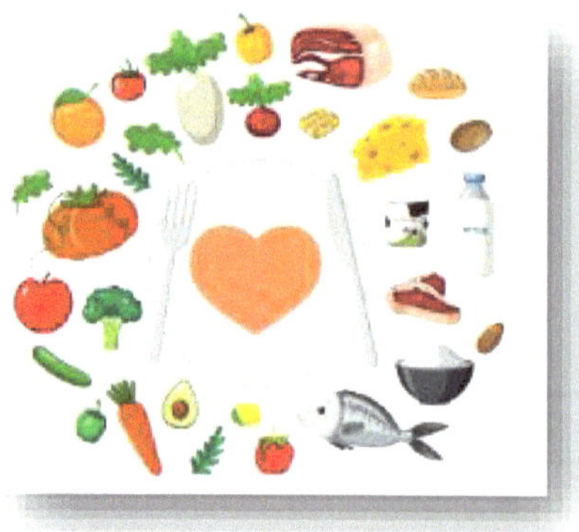

- Consume a variety of foods from all the food groups.
- Extra calories should come from nutritious foods, such as low-fat meats and dairy products, fruits, vegetables and whole grain starches.
    - Examples of low-fat protein sources: chicken & turkey (white meat), fish, skim milk
    - Examples of heart-healthy fats: salmon, avocado, almonds, walnut, olive oil, flaxseed
    - Examples of whole grains: whole wheat or multigrain bread, wheat pasta, brown rice
- Avoid foods and drinks with a lot of added sugar. A high-sugar diet while breastfeeding can cause a yeast infection in mom and baby.
- If you feel your baby is bothered by a certain food you eat, stop eating that food for at least 3 days and try it again when your baby is older.

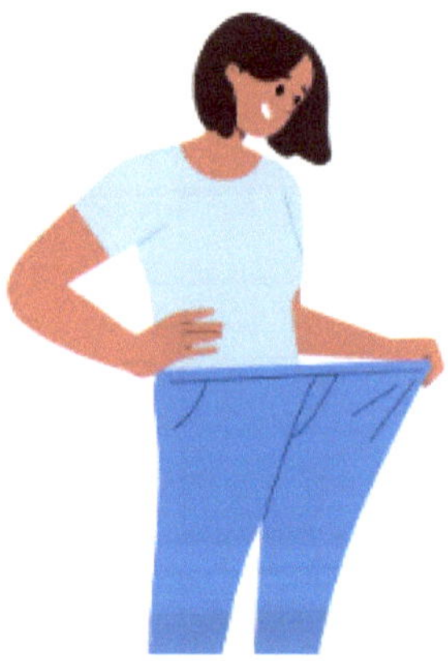

Weight Loss

- When combined with a healthy diet, breastfeeding can aid in weight loss after your baby is born.
- Do not try to lose weight until your milk supply is established so that you can make enough breast milk and you do not lose nutrients that your baby needs.
- Restricting calories to less than 1500-1800 calories per day can decrease milk supply and is not recommended.
- Once your milk supply is established, slow weight loss of 5 pounds per month is recommended.

Lactation Cookies

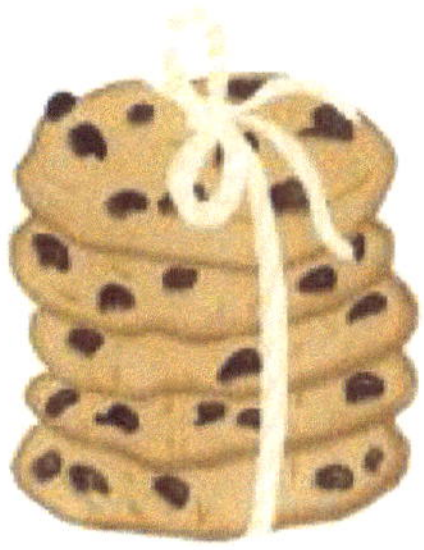

- Lactation cookies contain ingredients (oats, fenugreek, flaxseed, and Brewer's yeast) that are thought to improve breast milk production.
- There is no scientific evidence to support this, but they are safe and contain nutritious ingredients.
- Make sure you are drinking plenty of water with these cookies to avoid constipation.
- Make sure you read food labels to avoid consuming too many calories from these cookies as you are trying to lose weight.

Foods and Items to Avoid

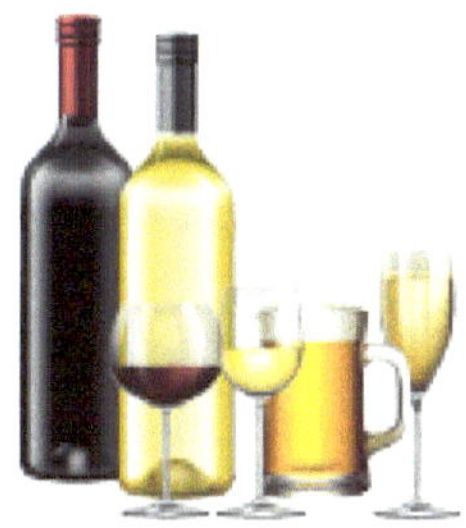

- When breastfeeding, try to wait until your baby is at least 3 months old until you drink alcohol.
- Avoid alcohol for at least 2 hours before you plan to breastfeed. If you need to pump while consuming alcohol, you should dump that milk.

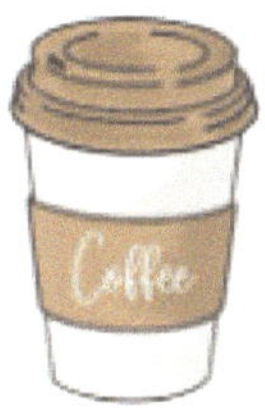

- Limit drinks with caffeine (such as coffee, tea, soda, energy drinks) to no more than 2-3 cups per day. Too much caffeine can make your baby fussy and irritable and can interrupt their sleep.
- Avoid herbal teas, remedies and supplements.
- Discuss with your doctor before taking Fenugreek products to make sure if does not interact with any other medications you might be taking.

Fish

- Fish is a great source of protein and omega-3 fatty acids, which are essential for your baby's development. Salmon, sardines, light canned tuna, pollock and catfish are good sources.
- Avoid fish with high mercury levels. This includes shark, swordfish, king mackerel, and tile fish.
- Limit lower mercury fish and shellfish to 12 ounces per week and albacore tuna to 6 ounces per week.

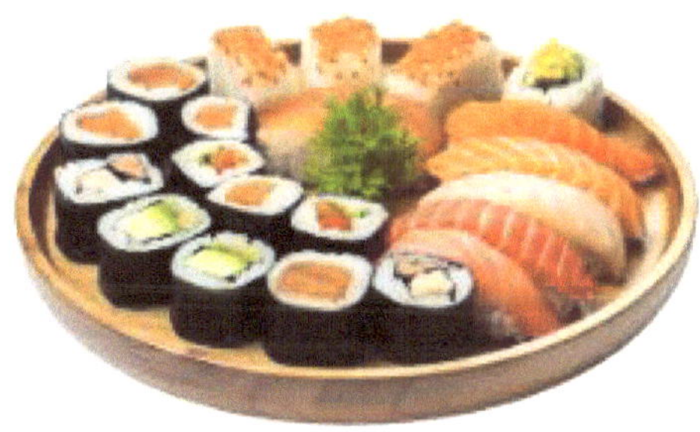

Special Needs for Vegetarian and Vegan Moms

- Vegan and vegetarian moms need to get protein, iron, calcium, and Vitamin B12 from different sources.
- Plant sources of protein are soy products and meat substitutes, legumes, lentils, nuts, seeds, and whole grains. Eggs and dairy are other protein options.
- Good sources of iron include lentils, enriched cereals, leafy green vegetables, peas, and dried fruit, such as raisins. To help your body absorb iron, eat iron-rich foods with foods high in vitamin C, such as citrus fruits.
- Good sources of calcium include dairy products and dark green vegetables. Other options are calcium-enriched and -fortified products, such as juices, cereals, soy milk, soy yogurt, and tofu.

Food Allergies in Your Baby

- In rare cases a breastfeeding baby may develop a food allergy to foods the mother is eating. Talk to your pediatrician if you think your baby has a food allergy before you make any diet changes.
- The most common foods that cause allergies are dairy products, soy products, wheat and eggs.
- Less common foods that cause allergies include fish, nuts, peanuts or corn.
- A baby could develop an allergy to any food you eat.
- Keeping a food diary of symptoms along with what you eat might help you know which foods are causing the problem.
- Removing the suspected foods from your diet by carefully reading all food labels should solve the problem but it may take 4-6 weeks for the infant's symptoms to resolve.
- A visit with a registered dietitian experienced with food allergies may help you plan your diet.

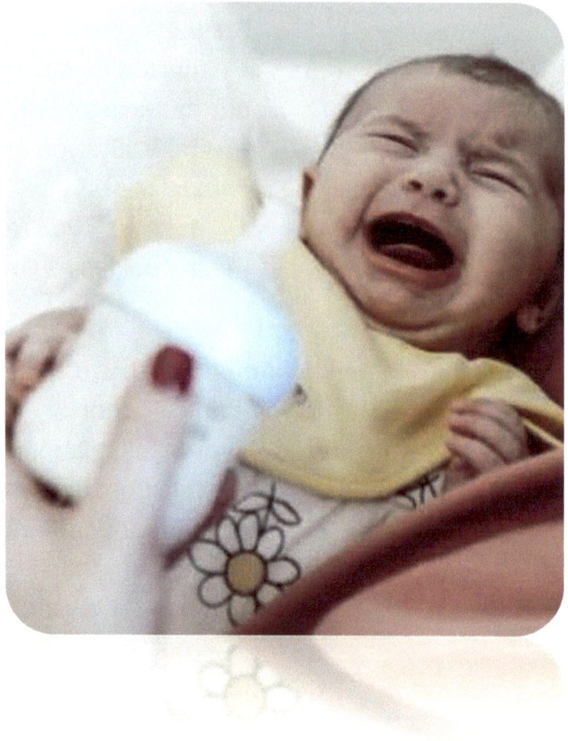

Signs of a food allergy reaction in babies:

- Localized Hives
- One or two episodes of vomiting
- Itchy, watery eyes
- Runny nose
- Itching
- Local skin redness

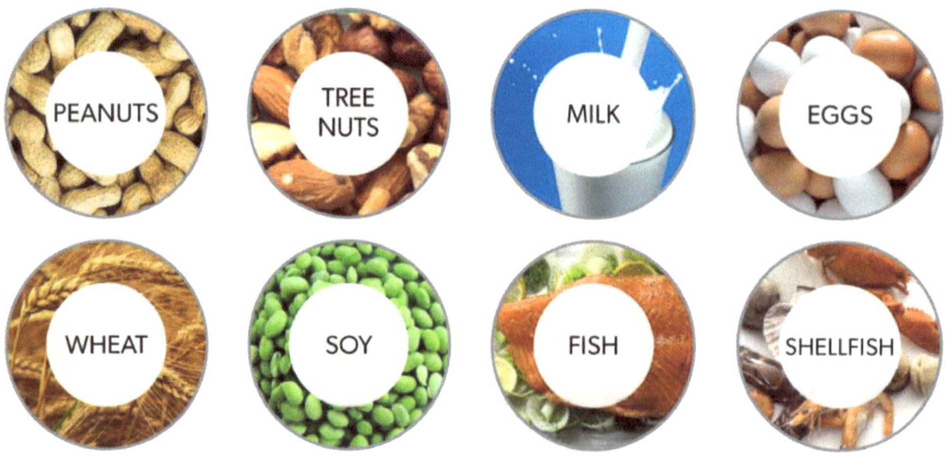

meet BRIDGET

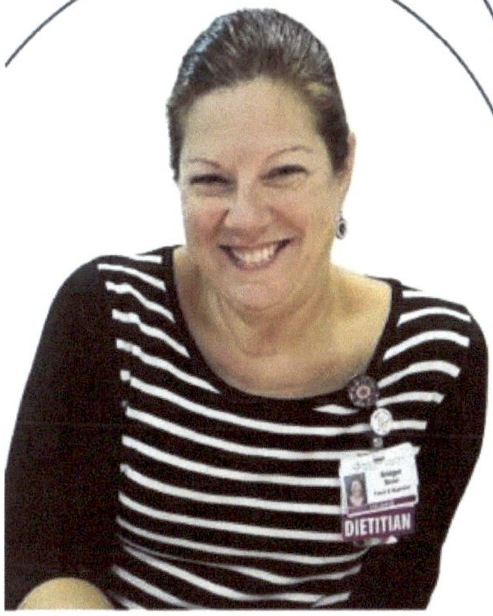

Hi there! My name is Bridget Storm, and I'm a CNSC with a passion for mentoring aspiring clinicians. I've been in critical care and nutrition support for 17 years and I absolutely love it! I enjoy writing and creating and I'm always looking for ways to learn more and expand my knowledge.

ACKNOWLEDGEMENTS

As the author of this training guide, I want to express my heartfelt thanks to you for taking the time to engage with my work. Your interest in learning and dedication to advancing your NICU nutrition support skills are deeply appreciated. Writing this guide has been a rewarding experience and knowing that it might assist you on your career journey brings me great satisfaction. Thank you for your support and for considering this guide as a resource.

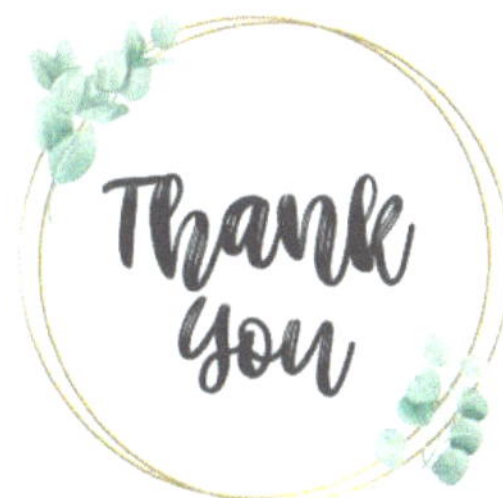

I would like to thank my former NICU mentor and champion, Dr. Deb Tuttle. Your dedication and support for progressing the nutrition care of this special population inspires me to continue to push for excellence. I cherish the guidance you have provided me over the years, and I aspire to follow in your footsteps!

I'd also like to thank my friend Katie Roche for encouraging me to write this training guide – and for always sharing my social media posts to help spread awareness for my products.

Finally, I would like to extend my deepest thanks to my husband, David Storm, for his patience with my long hours and his support of "The Side Hustle".